ETHICAL DIMENSIONS

IN THE HEALTH PROFESSIONS

ETHICAL DIMENSIONS

IN THE HEALTH PROFESSIONS

THIRD EDITION

Ruth Purtilo, PhD

Director and C. C. and Mabel L. Criss Professor
Creighton University Center for Health Policy and Ethics
Omaha, Nebraska

W.B. SAUNDERS COMPANY
A Division of Harcourt Brace & Company
Philadelphia   London   Toronto   Montreal   Sydney   Tokyo

W.B. SAUNDERS COMPANY

A *Division of Harcourt Brace & Company*

The Curtis Center
Independence Square West
Philadelphia, Pennsylvania 19106

Library of Congress Cataloging-in-Publication Data

Purtilo, Ruth B.
    Ethical dimensions in the health professions / Ruth Purtilo. —
3rd ed.
      p.   cm.
    Includes bibliographical references and index.
    ISBN 0-7216-7799-1
    1. Medical ethics.   2. Medicine—Moral and ethical aspects.
I. Title.
    [DNLM: 1. Ethics, Medical. W 50 P986e 1999]
    R724.P82   1999
    174'.2—dc21
    DNLM/DLC
                                 98-44276

ETHICAL DIMENSIONS IN THE HEALTH PROFESSIONS   ISBN 0-7216-7799-1

Printed in the United States of America

Last digit is the print number: 9   8   7   6   5   4   3   2   1

For
Henry Lemon, MD
and
Polly Cerasoli, PT

I am deeply grateful for
the support they offered me
over the years;
I am instructed by their
compassion and commitment
to the high ethical standards of their profession.

Preface

Life-prolonging technologies, assisted suicide, and the promises and cautions regarding new genetic and reproductive technologies are in the news daily as this third edition goes to press. Worldwide the population is growing older, the gap between the rich and the poor in their access to basic health care is growing, and the ravages of the AIDS epidemic are well into their second decade. Infectious diseases such as tuberculosis, always a scourge in some parts of the world, are on the increase in the United States and elsewhere. The organization and institutional dimensions of health care are changing worldwide too: for instance, in the United States, "managed care" is a relatively recent attempt to contain escalating health care costs through a radical reorganization of the delivery and financing of health care services. Similar experiments are being launched in Europe and Asia.

Each of these themes and many others provide challenges for health professionals, that group of people in any society who have chosen to commit their lives and careers to the maintenance of health and the amelioration of the physical, emotional, and spiritual suffering caused by disease or injury. This textbook is expressly *for* them, the goal being to provide ethical tools they can use to build understanding, resolve problems, and take full advantage of their skills to improve the lot of patients, the community, and themselves. The tone is practical throughout, not a book for philosophers but for people on the front lines of health care decision making. The textbook also is written *by* them, the first edition having been co-authored by Dr. Christine Cassel, a physician, and myself, a physical therapist. (During the updating of the subsequent two single-authored editions my everyday work has reflected my career movement more fully into my professional role as an ethicist in the health care setting.) In each edition the content has taken shape as a result of the privilege to work directly with patients or health professions students, practitioners, and administrators across a broad spectrum of disciplines in several parts of the world. The gift of these patients, other health professionals, and health administrators to the reader of this textbook is that they have allowed Dr. Cassel and me to glean insight from their experiences and their own willingness to grapple with perplexing ethical dimensions of health care. They have also taught us, and can teach the reader, about the vast store of personal and professional resources available for effectively resolving ethical issues.

The third edition builds on the previous two, the foundation stones being those enduring concerns that have supported the need for professional ethics and ethical professionals since the beginnings of health care. It also builds on my abiding conviction that health professionals can and should assume a strategic position to help shape the contours of today's health care environment so that it embraces and protects cherished social values. The weight of responsibility for constructing or reinforcing high ethical standards must be shouldered by all health professionals, not just doctors or nurses, and not turned over to philosophers, theologians, administrators, or policy makers (distinguishing us today, I might add, from our forebears in the health professions).

Some dramatic changes in the health care educational environment since the release of the first, and to some extent the second, edition have influenced this new edition. Overall I have witnessed an increasing awareness by educators that patients and the larger society expect all health professionals to be informed about the ethics of the issues and to be moral agents in helping to address them. In response, administrators and teachers in professional education have implemented professional ethics course requirements, ethics seminars, and continuing education opportunities. Furthermore, educators skillfully have woven ethics theory and practice into the very fabric of the student's educational experience rather than limiting it to one ethics course. With these changes, it is not surprising that there has been a proliferation of written and on-line resources for new students and life-long learners alike. In short, I have observed a promising increase in sophistication and interest in professional ethics and in a commitment to providing educational experiences geared to improving knowledge and skills in this area. My goal in preparing this updated and expanded edition has been to reflect these positive changes by offering an instrument that educators can use to meet the changing needs of the classroom, seminar, and self-learning settings while maintaining the no-frills approach that has helped assure the book's utility during the past decade.

WHAT'S NEW IN THIS EDITION

With these encouraging considerations as guideposts, the third edition of *Ethical Dimensions in the Health Professions* includes a greatly *expanded but to-the-point section on ethics theories and approaches*. Some have been introduced into the professional ethics arena only in recent years, but the new generation of health professionals should have the benefit of becoming familiar with them. *The problem-solving method is refined* as a result of welcome input from many readers of the first two editions. The third edition takes both traditional and emerging roles of health professionals seriously: it addresses the health professional as *an individual moral agent* (including one's moral agency as a student) and as *a moral participant in team decisions*. The reader also has an opportunity to learn about how he or she is shaped by organizational structures and can be effective as *a framer of ethical policies and practices* in the institutions of health care. Finally, an updated section on health professionals as citizens provides new insight into how one's professional expertise and commitment can provide guidance for one's role as *a contributor to the common good in the broader community*.

As in previous editions, the textbook does not assume that the reader has engaged in any previous formal study of ethics. For those who have, the first chapters may seem elementary, but scanning them should provide a quick and helpful review. The scope is broad. Those wanting more rigorous study in a particular topic fortunately will find ample materials available, both on-line and in hard copy. For those wishing additional work in basic philosophical, theological, or other theories and approaches to ethical issues, there are excellent texts and courses, including an increasing number of short-term intensive courses offered during summer months. *Ethical Dimensions in the Health Professions* is a basic map and backpack of supplies for what I trust will be a lifelong and generative journey of professional ethics exploration, reflection, and effective professional judgment and action. This journey is, I believe, the key to finding self-fulfillment in professional life. Once begun, the reader will find many other trekkers to walk and talk with along the way, each compelled and all connected by wanting to help foster the best type of health care possible.

Ruth Purtilo

Acknowledgments
Edition Three

The first edition of this book was co-authored. It grew out of Christine Cassel's and my separate experiences as health professionals and students of ethics and out of our mutual concerns about the ethical dimensions of health care.

Christine, now a leading geriatrics specialist, educator, and administrator continues to make significant contributions to this important aspect of health professions practice and policy. Although she has not retained her position as a co-author, readers familiar with her work will recognize her ideas and insights woven into the very warp and woof of this edition.

The idea for the first edition began after each of us had attended a summer seminar on ethical issues for medical practitioners sponsored by the National Endowment for the Humanities and taught by William May. The opportunity to step out of our everyday professional involvements to reflect on the ethical quandaries of working in health care teams was the beginning of an approach that more fully allowed us to integrate philosophy and the practice of our professions, bringing greater fulfillment in each. I know I convey Christine's gratitude as well as my own to Dr. May for his lively, sincere, and thoughtful teaching and to our colleagues in the seminars for their stimulation and support in wrestling with the issues.

The field of professional ethics continues to grow and become richer. Thus, it is impossible to acknowledge everyone who has made significant contributions to this and previous editions of the book through their writing and thinking, story telling and reflection, and considered action on the front lines of health care practice.

If anyone deserves special mention it is the health professions students I have had the opportunity to teach and learn from during the life of this book: at the University of Nebraska Medical Center; at the Karolinska Institute in Stockholm, Sweden; The Massachusetts General Hospital Institute of Health Professions, Boston, and Harvard Medical School; and Creighton University, Omaha, Nebraska.

JoAnn Maynard and Rita Nutty spent many hours typing, reviewing, proofing and in other ways preparing the manuscript for publication. They were a lifeline between the idea and reality of this edition, and I thank them for their able assistance. Mary Ellen Read worked with publishers and authors to secure permission to reprint material, and I am grateful for her help, also.

Over the years, I have benefited immeasurably from the able assistance of our editors and their staff at W.B. Saunders. I am especially grateful to Margaret Biblis for her support and substantive help in preparing the first and second editions and for encouraging me to prepare a third.

Notes to Instructors on Using This Edition

The core purpose of this book is to provide the tools for addressing common, everyday ethical issues in the health professions. I hope you will find it student *and* instructor user-friendly!

The six-step process of ethical decision-making (Chapter 5) is your most important organizing framework. I do not walk the student through each step every time a new case is examined, but you will find parts of the process mentioned in many chapters. In two chapters (8 and 10) I reinforce the whole process, step by step.

In general the other chapters of Section One, expanded from the first and second editions, can all be assigned or can be assigned discretely as building blocks for the use of the process:

THE SIX STEPS	BUILDING BLOCKS	CHAPTER
Step 1: Gather relevant information	*Case-driven approaches, care,* and *casuistry*—each highlights the importance of getting the story straight	2
Step 2: Identify the type of ethical problem	*Three prototypes*	3
Step 3: Analyze problem using ethics approaches	*Means, ends, principles, virtues*—ways conflicts can be thought through	4
Steps 4 and 5: Move to practical alternatives and action	These steps require knowledge, creativity, and courage	Life itself is the teacher
Step 6: Evaluation of results	Ethics: Reflecting on Morality	1

Other Instructional Tools

At the beginning of each chapter are

- Educational objectives for that chapter
- New terms introduced in that chapter (Note that those terms also appear in *italics* the first time the student encounters them.)
- A quick cross reference of key concepts used in that chapter and where each first appeared in the book

At the end of each chapter are questions for thought and discussion.

Ideas? Questions? Stories to tell? Write to me: rpurtilo@creighton.edu

Objectives

Through reading this book and discussing the Questions for Thought and Discussion, students will be able to

1. Increase their sensitivity to the influence of ethics in professional practice.
2. Become familiar with basic approaches and concepts widely used today in addressing ethical dimensions of professional practice and policy.
3. Recognize and cite examples of concrete ethical situations and problems in the health professions.
4. Gain insight into ethical situations and problems that are unique to their own profession, in contrast to those shared by a wide range of health professionals.
5. Apply a problem-solving method to ethical decision making.
6. Find resources useful for more in-depth study of professional ethics.

Contents

5 A Six-Step Process of Ethical Decision Making for You to Follow   79

SECTION TWO

Ethical Dimensions of Professional Roles   91

6 Surviving Student Life Ethically   93

GUIDE TO CASES AND STORIES IN TEXT

Introduction to Ethical Dimensions in the Health Professions

1

Morality and Ethics: What Are They and Why Do They Matter?

Objectives

The student should be able to:

- Define morality and ethics and distinguish between the two.
- Describe three moralities health professionals must integrate into their own moral life.
- Identify some major sources of moral beliefs in Western societies.
- Distinguish between an ethical issue and ethical problem.
- List three ways ethics is useful in everyday professional practice.
- Describe what material cooperation entails.
- Identify some mechanisms available to protect the personal moral convictions of health professionals.

New Terms and Ideas You Will Encounter in This Chapter

Morality	Ethics	Conscience
Values	Ethicists	Material cooperation
Duties	Ethics committees	State interest
Personal morality	Moral judgments	Licensing laws
Societal morality	Ethical issue	Moral repugnance
Group morality	Ethical problem	

Introduction

Your adventure into the world of health care ethics begins with a story. Throughout this text you will meet patients, health professionals, families, and others who are facing challenges posed by their situations and the health care environment. Their stories illustrate the types of ethical issues you yourself may face as a caregiver, a patient, or a family member. The underlying ethical themes in the stories are woven into the very fabric of health care.

Our first story is about Mr. and Mrs. Harvey and the health care system into which they are catapulted following his stroke.

THE STORY OF MR. AND MRS. HARVEY

Mr. Harvey, who is 61 years old, recently made a momentous decision: He will retire next year from his position as a high school mathematics teacher in the small town where he has taught for 30 years. Mr. Harvey's retirement salary will be somewhat less than if he waited until he was 65, but he and his wife want to spend time traveling.

JANUARY 6

During the past few weeks, excited about the decision they have made, the Harveys have begun planning a six-week cross country trip for the following June. Two days ago, however, Mr. Harvey complained of a severe dizzy spell. During dinner he suddenly began to mumble in nonsense syllables. Peas dribbled from one corner of his mouth, and Mrs. Harvey noticed that the right side of his face was drooping. Mr. Harvey had a confused and frightened expression on his face; he shrugged his left shoulder as if to ask, "What's happening?" Alice, his wife, jumped up, and Mr. Harvey too tried to stand up. Before she could reach him, he had fallen to the floor. He was taken to the emergency department of the hospital, where a diagnosis of cerebral vascular accident (stroke) was made.

The physician assistant on duty examined him with the help of several nurses and called the case manager for the health plan the Harveys subscribed to through the local school district. Mrs. Harvey listened as the physician assistant talked convincingly about the need to admit Mr. Harvey to the hospital. He asked Alice Harvey to sign informed consent, insurance, and other forms and began to prepare Mr. Harvey for admission to the hospital.

Mrs. Harvey felt tears welling up in her. When a nurse put an arm across Alice's shoulder and said, "I'm sorry," Alice began to weep. The nurse offered to get Alice a drink of water and guided her to a chair while explaining what would happen next.

JANUARY 15

After several days in the intensive care unit, Mr. Harvey was transferred to the medical unit. This morning the physician told Alice that Mr. Harvey was "stabilized" and would be going home soon. "Home!" Alice gasped. "How can we possibly manage at home? He can't talk, can't walk, can't go to the bathroom alone!" The physician explained that the Harveys would be visited by a home care nurse and for some time (depending on his progress) by a physical therapist. A home health aid would also visit them. He reminded her that Mr. Harvey was improving, and while it was impossible to predict how much he would finally improve, everyone was hopeful.

FEBRUARY 15

At home his right arm and hand regained function so that he could almost dress himself. He is righthanded but as yet could not hold a pencil. He couldn't walk because of spasticity of the right leg, although the spasticity seemed at times to be subsiding. He suffered from expressive aphasia; he had a limited vocabulary but increasingly caught himself when he used a wrong word. Because of this progress the case manager authorized another six weeks of therapy and other interventions. Speech therapy was initiated.

Mrs. Harvey was understandably anxious but very supportive throughout the entire ordeal, encouraging her husband toward as much independence as possible and offering support when needed. Mr. Harvey's brother made some adjustments in the Harveys' home to accommodate Mr. Harvey's impaired state.

TODAY (APRIL 1)

The several health professionals working with Mr. Harvey have grown attached to him and Alice. They have rejoiced with every sign of progress and have struggled with him through the frustration and depression that accompany such a catastrophe. But the health professionals are now faced with a difficult situation. Another treatment review is due. Understandably, when no further progress can be shown, authorization for his treatments (and therefore the reimbursements for them) will be discontinued.

Anyone who works with stroke patients knows, however, that this creates a delicate situation. The rate of "progress" is not always constant. It may be marked by periods of rapid improvement interspersed with other periods of almost no perceptible change (plateaus). If the patient ceases to receive maintenance treatments during these plateau periods, a dramatic loss in functioning often occurs. Yet many insurance plans make little or no allowance for these plateau periods, and treatment usually is discontinued. The patient must regress to the point at which a symptom becomes acute before treatment can be reinstituted. In short, while progress eventually does end, the failure to allow for a plateau period often results in the patient's being prematurely discontinued from treatment altogether. This is precisely the challenge facing the health professionals who have been treating Mr. Harvey.

Mr. Harvey's speech and progress toward ambulation have plateaued. Every sign indicates to the health professionals that he will realize more improvement if his treatment is not discontinued at this critical juncture, but the outcomes measurements (by which his health plan will continue to authorize further treatment) do not fall within a range that would justify further reimbursement. The health professionals know that continued payments for treatment depend on their report of his progress. What should they do?

- Should they tell a lie and report that Mr. Harvey continues to make daily progress, so that he will be less likely to lose an opportunity for almost certain further progress?
- Should they tell the truth and let Mr. Harvey be discontinued from treatment at this time?
- Are there alternatives to an either-or solution to this perplexing problem?
- Should they get involved in trying to change the insurance company policies that put them in this difficult bind in the first place?

Suppose *you* are treating Mr. Harvey. You probably will ask yourself if Mr. Harvey should continue to be treated even if it means not exactly telling the truth on a report. Questions with a broader outlook might occur as well. For instance, is it fair to continue treating him if you are not prepared to make a similar defense for all patients in a comparable situation? Or, an even broader scope may be encompassed: Are you as a health professional responsible for trying to change the system so that such situations do not occur and you can more easily give patients what you think they need? Take a minute to jot down what you think are the most important issues in the Harveys' story, whether or not they are suggested in the above text:

_____

_____

_____

_____

Responses to these concerns and questions are not to be found in the textbooks that deal with the technical skills of your chosen field. You are beginning to use your understanding of morality and how ethics figures into your professional life if you are thinking about what would be *right or wrong* conduct for you in this situation and *why*; what your *duties* are to everyone involved, and what your (and everyone else's) *rights* are; the type of *character traits* you want to preserve; or what constitutes *fairness* for all patients in similar situations. These considerations may even make you think about what type of society you want to help build.

MORALITY AND MORAL VALUES

When the moral life or morality is mentioned, you might think of what you were told to do or not to do as a child. That *is* a part of morality. But morality is a much richer idea than that. From the earliest societies onward people have established guidelines designed to preserve the very fabric of their society. Taken collectively, these guidelines are a society's morality.

Morality, then, is concerned with relations between people and how, ultimately, they can best live in peace and harmony. The goal of morality is to protect a high quality of life for an individual or for the community as a whole. We all try to act in accordance with morality in our everyday lives. It makes things go better and gives more meaning to life. Morality is made up of a lot of values and duties based on beliefs that people take for granted most of the time.

Values is the language that has evolved to talk about objects or things a person holds dear. An apt example is life. You most likely hold life dear (i.e., value it) because without it you cannot really do anything else. Moral values, then, describe certain qualities that constitute "a good life" from the perspective of how persons can live in peace and harmony with others.

Duties is a language that has evolved to describe actions in response to claims on you that are either self-imposed or imposed by others. Moral duties describe certain actions required of you if you are to play your part in building a society in which persons can live in peace and harmony with others.

As a child you acquired parts of your morality from parents and friends, from reading and television, from your religious teaching, and in school. Behavior was modified when knowingly or unknowingly you did something outside of what you had been taught is right and were punished or shamed by others for what you did (or failed to do). One of the primary tasks of growing up is to internalize or personalize aspects of the morality that have come from the various sources. In fact, there is a whole area of study in psychology called "moral development," which deals with theories of how and why persons become the types of moral beings they are.

Take a moment to think about the sources that have led to your own moral beliefs and complete the following two questions:

1. Who or what have been the five most important influences on your understanding of right and wrong?

   _____

   _____

   _____

   _____

   _____

2. Name three people whom you admire. Try to state what it is about them that makes them admirable. They can be people you know personally or only by reputation.

   _____

   _____

   _____

Your answers can be personal reference points for you as you read on about morality.

Morality informs many decisions in your everyday experience, but usually you are so used to moving through life in accordance with its values and duties that you have little conscious awareness of it. In short, it is safe to say that morality is habitual, shaping the character of individuals and communities without them even realizing it.

As a student entering the health professions you must reckon with at least three subgroups of morality: your personal morality, societal morality, and the morality of the health professions and its institutions. Fortunately there are large areas of overlap. In fact, almost everyone experiences the moral life as a whole, whether as an individual among family members or friends, as a citizen, or as a professional, because the sources of moral belief usually derive from similar understandings of value and right and wrong, and large groups of society interpret their dictates similarly.

Personal Morality

Personal morality is made up of the values and duties you have adopted as relevant. You may recognize them as customs, laws, rules, beliefs, or simply "the way things always were done in my family." They influenced your judgment about Mr. Harvey when you read his story. Saints and moral heroes have so fully personalized what they learned that they can stand alone in their convictions when opportunities for wrongdoing arise and make decisions that others admire because they are exemplary. Everyone has a personal morality, however imperfectly internalized. One task you face as a health professional is to try to understand the personal morality of your patients, clients, colleagues, and others with whom you come in contact. Without sensitivity to the differences between your own and their personal moral beliefs and habits you will not be able to communicate or work together effectively. Before proceeding, try to think of four or five things you would call a part of your own personal morality (e.g., lying is wrong; I should be kind to myself and others; everyone deserves respect).

1. _____
2. _____
3. _____
4. _____
5. _____

Some of your answers probably came from the persons or other influences you listed as sources of your own moral beliefs. Over time you have adopted them as your own.

If you have time, compare your list with a friend. Are there large areas of overlap? Usually there are because you also participate together in a larger societal morality.

Societal Morality

Large components of personal morality represent a common denominator of shared belief about values and duties called *societal morality*. Sometimes they are culturally, ethnically, class-, or geographically generated. Almost always they spring from deeper religious and philosophic beliefs about humans and their relationship with God (or the gods in some cultures) or with each other. In the United States the founding legislators, who had risked crossing oceans and leaving behind almost every security, tried to capture the common denominator of their societal morality in a slogan stating that all "are created equal" and that therefore everyone should have an equal chance at "life, liberty and the pursuit of happiness." One characteristic of a democratic society in good working order is that everyone engages in critiquing and refining morality (e.g., laws, customs, and other moral components of the society) to keep it on course.

Almost always some tensions exist between personal and societal morality. These tensions are played out in large societal debates with individuals and groups taking sides. Two health care–related debates today deal with the morality of abortion and physician-assisted suicide. The use of the environment, the status of immigrants, and taxation are examples of other debates. Can you name another? _____

Group Morality: The Health Professions and Their Institutions

Everyone except perhaps the most resolute recluse joins or is swept into one or more subgroups of society by virtue of being a member of a church, a club, an organization, or other group. This can be termed *group morality*. One such subgroup, the health professions, has some moral values and duties that do not apply to others in society. To help inform you about the special values and duties of the health professional, you will be introduced to traditional oaths and codes of ethics as well as modern customs and standards of professional practice throughout your professional preparation. A careful study of them (along with reading this book and other ethics resource materials and observing your role models) will highlight aspects of this morality. Since the Hippocratic Oath is so well known, it is included here for you to read carefully (see page 10). Which aspects of this ancient moral oath taken by doctors still seem applicable today? What are its shortcomings?

Today, in modern bureaucratized society, much of the morality of the health professions is embedded in the policies, customs, and practices of

HIPPOCRATIC OATH

I swear by Apollo the Physician, by Aesculapius, Hygeia, and Panacea, and all the gods and goddesses, making them my witnesses, that I will fulfill according to my ability and judgment this oath and this covenant:

To hold him who has taught me this art as equal to my parents and to live my life in partnership with him, and if he is in need of money to give him a share of mine, and to regard his offspring as equal to my brothers in male lineage and to teach them this art—if they desire to learn it—without fee and covenant; to give a share of precepts and oral instruction and all the other learning to my sons and to the sons of him who has instructed me and to pupils who have signed the covenant and have taken an oath according to the medical law, but to no one else.

I will apply dietetic measures for the benefit of the sick according to my ability and judgment; I will keep them from harm and injustice.

I will neither give a deadly drug to anybody if asked for it, nor will I make a suggestion to this effect. Similarly I will not give to a woman an abortive remedy. In purity and holiness I will guard my life and my art.

I will not use the knife, not even on sufferers from stone, but will withdraw in favor of such men as are engaged in this work.

Whatever houses I may visit, I will come for the benefit of the sick, remaining free of all intentional injustice, of all mischief and in particular of sexual relations with both female and male persons, be they free or slaves.

What I may see or hear in the course of the treatment or even outside of the treatment in regard to the life of men, which on no account one must spread abroad, I will keep to myself holding such things shameful to be spoken about.

If I fulfill this oath and do not violate it, may it be granted to me to enjoy life and art, being honored with fame among all men for all time to come; if I transgress it and swear falsely, may the opposite of all this be my lot.

From Edelstein, L. 1943. The Hippocratic Oath: Text, translation and interpretation. *Bulletin of the History of Medicine* 2(suppl):3. © Johns Hopkins University Press, Baltimore, Md. Reprinted with permission.

health care *institutions*. For instance, you probably have an honor code in your educational institution. And when you reach the clinical years you will become familiar with policies specific to the institutions where you complete your professional preparation. Federal and state laws embody and codify moral values and duties that should govern individual and institutional conduct. For instance, laws about informed consent, confidentiality, and the competence required of persons working as professionals are based on moral values and duties the professional has to society.

Occasionally the values and duties of a person come into conflict with the morality of a subgroup she or he has joined. For instance, the Christian Reformation in the 1500s took place when the personal morality of some religious leaders came into conflict with the customs and patterns of moral conduct in the institution of the church. The famous statement "Here I stand. I can do no other" exemplifies the moral breaking point persons sometimes reach. It is attributed to reformist Martin Luther as he nailed 95 objections to the official church morality regarding a practice called "indulgences" to the door of All Saints Church in Wittenberg, Germany. In health care today the accepted professional morality may conflict with the belief and conscience of a professional's personal morality. Abortion is one issue that has caused deep consternation for some health professionals because of their personal morality. Many hospitals and clinics have accepted an interpretation of professional morality that commits the institution to enabling medically safe abortions to women under the conditions detailed in *Roe v. Wade* and other law. Protections of personal morality built into the professional morality are described at the end of this chapter in the case of abortion and some other important social issues. In another example, such protection is not assured: Some health professionals object to treating gay patients with AIDS because of a personal morality that rejects a gay lifestyle. No protection of personal morality of this type today overrides the professional duty to provide "due care" to everyone whose symptoms and other signs require intervention.[1] The predicament that the health professionals found themselves in regarding Mr. Harvey's care presents a big problem because it is safe to assume that most of them would find it personally wrong to lie. At the same time, some of them probably are considering it because the institutional policies seem unfair.

Summary

In its barest form, morality keeps individuals and groups directed toward behaviors and values that assure they can sustain themselves. Beyond that, the positive goal of thriving in a harmonious environment presents itself as a possibility.

I like to think of the path of morality as one that individuals and groups can follow with ease and confidence most of the time because of good customs, laws, traditions, and other markers that have been posted. For an individual the path will be the most trouble free when her or his personal, societal, and group moralities are identical. However, philosophers, psychologists, and others who have thought about such things remind us that constant vigilance and frequent reflection are needed to keep us clear about the relevance of our values and duties. Some dimensions of and standards for the morally good life never change, but morality itself is context dependent insofar as it is useful only in a specific time and place. The question then is, Is the accepted morality fitting for *this* time and *this* place in history (my own or the human community's)? When the fittingness disappears, the experience is akin to stubbing a toe on a rock in your path. You lose your balance. It hurts. It makes you take notice. You probably noted that even in the description of personal, social, and group moralities I raised the possibility of problems and conflicts that could arise at each step of the way.

Ethics is the discipline that provides a language, some methods, and guidelines for studying the components of personal, societal, and group morality to create a better path for yourself and others.

ETHICS: REFLECTING ON MORALITY

Ethics is a systematic reflection on morality: "systematic" because it is a discipline that uses special methods and approaches to examine moral situations and "reflection" because it consciously calls into question assumptions about existing components of moralities that fall into the category of habits, customs, or traditions. Originally the systems of analysis were developed as parts of philosophy and theology. Today other disciplines have added to the number and types of tools that are useful for such a task. (For an elaboration, see Chapter 2, pages 30–37).

Ethics, using the inherent dignity of human life and deep respect for all life and the environment as the standard, asks, What do dignity and respect demand in terms of response from others? Following are some of the most important subsequent questions:

- Do our present values, behaviors, and character traits pass the test of further examination when measured against this standard?
- In situations where conflicts arise, which values, duties, and other guidelines are the most important and why?
- When new situations present uncertainty, what aspects of present moralities will most reliably guide individuals and societies on a sustainable path for survival and thriving?
- What new thinking is needed in such situations and why?

Ethicists have as their primary career activity the work of ethics. They help to clarify values, duties, and other aspects of morality in specific situations. (Medical ethicists or health care ethicists specialize in areas of health care.) They work as consultants in the design of policies and practices. The ethicist also consults with persons or groups who are faced with situations of high moral uncertainty or who are experiencing conflict between competing values and duties. In many institutions today *ethics committees* serve much the same purpose and often include ethicists as well as thoughtful professionals and lay people.

But ethics is not the work of ethicists or ethics committees only. Ethics work is a fundamental part of the life of every thoughtful citizen and takes specific forms when someone assumes a special role such as health professional. And so as this book proceeds, I am assuming that each of you is learning to become a role ethicist, capable of analyzing morality issues within your role as a health professional.

Moral Judgments, Ethical Issues, and Ethical Problems

I suggested that ethics comes to the rescue when you "stub your toe" on your walk down the moral path of life. The process of making an assessment and arriving at a conclusion in such moments is called *a moral judgment*. The philosopher David Hume speculated about the conditions that should help to assure correct moral judgments such as getting all the facts, being impartial, and trying to think about whether you would be willing to generalize your conclusion to affect everyone in similar situations.[2]

An *ethical issue* is any situation you believe may have important moral challenges embedded in it that you want to identify. For instance, in the 1950s when the idea of organ transplantation began to be discussed, speculation began immediately that an ethical issue was present because the prospect that another person's (or an animal's) body part would be inserted into a human being raised serious questions about the morality of this type of activity. Many asked, Does it support a type of human community that honors cherished values and duties? Aren't we playing God?

What are some aspects of the idea of human organ transplantation that makes it an ethical issue?

_____

_____

If you answered that some types of transplantation could save the life of persons who otherwise would have died, you would be correct. Having reflected on the situation you could conclude with confidence that the moral value of human life is honored through this procedure. If you answered, I'm not sure that the costs involved for this type of treatment justify the expense to society, or Healthy animals should not be sacrificed to extend the life span of a human being, or Some types of transplantation may have such poor results that more harm than good will be done to the patient, you would be raising areas of concern about the morality of the procedure that others raised (and continue to raise).

An *ethical problem* is a situation that you have reason to believe has serious negative implications regarding cherished moral values and duties and that will pose extremely difficult choices for persons who want to help support high moral standards. The categories of ethical problems faced by health professionals, patients, and society in the health care environment are discussed in Chapter 4.

The Moral and Ethical Thing to Do

It is common to hear someone say, "That's the moral and ethical thing to do." You will hear the terms "moral" and "ethical" used interchangeably. I suggest you use them more purposefully, however, because after what you have just learned, that phrase should have more meaning for you. The "moral thing to do" means that the traditions, customs, laws, and other markers that an individual and society call upon for habitual moral guidance allow them to proceed with confidence in their course of action. Conversely, the "ethical thing to do" means that the course of action that would be taken in the everyday moral walk of life has been reflected on and your moral judgment dictates that it still seems the right thing to do. Fortunately, most situations allow you to act both morally and ethically!

Using Ethics in Practical Situations Involving Morality

The scholarly discipline of ethics has always been interesting from the point of view that its subject matter has immediate relevance for everyday life. Aristotle and others in the classical Greek era called ethics "practical philosophy." In the next chapters you will see how the concepts and methods of ethics are tools to help you in the analysis of moral problems, in the resolution of moral conflicts, and in keeping your actions consistent with high moral standards.

Analysis

Analysis of morality allows you to stand back and identify categories of issues and problems as well as to delineate which of the aspects of morality are involved in any situation. One type of analysis is the process you engage in when two parts of your own morality collide: "I shouldn't lie to my spouse, but the truth will be bitter, and I shouldn't hurt her either." We already have considered some examples of how your personal set of values and your society's or subgroup's values could collide. Martin Luther had to analyze his own morality and his church's when he made his decision. The medieval physician Galen fled Rome during the plague. He analyzed his personal morality and decided he had to flee on behalf of his wife and children whose lives he knew were threatened by the plague, but all of his life he had nightmares about his "failure" because he believed he had also abandoned his patients. In other words, his belief about his personal and professional duties collided. The analysis of situations allows one to know *why* there are psychological and other practical consequences of proposed action. Therefore, analysis leads to knowledge that can inform action.

Resolution

Another practical use of ethical reflection is to actually resolve conflict. This goes beyond solely analyzing a situation and categorizing it. In other words, the knowledge base of analysis is complemented by a process that works toward resolution. One approach to finding resolution is to try to build consensus among the various concerned parties (e.g., yourself, patients, families, the institution). This requires that those involved have analyzed the situation, are willing to hear everyone's point of view, will assist others in clarifying their own view, and are willing to facilitate the building of morally acceptable courses of action. Some ethics approaches focus on how to resolve issues when there is no consensus or when consensus does not seem to fully address the moral challenges embedded in the situation.

Action

Purposive action can stem from analysis and successful work toward resolution. The health professionals involved with Mr. Harvey's potential discharge from their care are looking for an action guide. The party responsible for putting ethics into action is the *moral agent*.

Summary

Today the recognition that ethics can be used for analysis, for resolution of complex situations, and ultimately as a guide for action has led to a resurgence of interest in ethics in various practical contexts. Health care ethics is one such area of applied ethics.

Ethics Research

To understand exactly what is important for ethical analysis, resolution, and action in the health care context, studies are conducted to identify behaviors and beliefs of people or groups around ethical issues or ethical problems. Social scientists (anthropologists, sociologists, and psychologists) are among the most active in this area of research. For instance, through research we now know that there are differences in cultural and ethnic groups regarding their understanding of and response to the Western European idea of informed consent. Such knowledge can help everyone to gauge the effectiveness of the mechanisms that have been developed to protect important values and duties. There is also continuing research on basic concepts of ethical approaches and theory. This pursuit is more in keeping with classical scholarship, which continues to enrich the whole discipline of ethics.

MORALITY—ETHICS AND FOLLOWING YOUR OWN CONSCIENCE

In the discussion so far, you have been introduced to how you can recognize the values and duties that make up your own morality as well as those with which you will be required to reckon in your activities as a professional and as a member of society. You have also begun your exploration into how ethics will help you when challenges to everyday morality arise. In this last section you will have an opportunity to think about institutional and social protections available to you as a professional when and if you encounter a situation (e.g., an instance or policy) that you believe compromises the dictates of your *conscience*.

> Sally Lim is one of the health professionals involved in Mr. Harvey's care. She is attending the patient evaluation conference called by the home health care coordinator to discuss what to do in relation to discontinuing Mr. Harvey. Sally assumes that the only option available to the home health care team is to discontinue him even though she is among those who believe most ardently that he could benefit from more of her interventions and those of other team members. She is prepared to express her difficulty with the reimbursement policy's unresponsiveness to patients like Mr. Harvey and her regret and anger that he cannot receive more therapy. She also plans to tell Mr. Harvey how she feels and to document in his clinical record something like the following: "My judgment is that this patient should not be discontinued at this time since his clinical profile is similar to that of many patients whose progress plateaus for a brief period but after which real progress is realized. Patient discontinued because utilization review recommends this course of action."
>
> The first part of the patient evaluation conference goes as Sally had imagined, everyone agreeing with her assessment of his clinical status. She is comfortable in stating her assumptions and expressing her feelings to the group. However, one of her colleagues, Nick, responds, "What we really *should* do is to lie about his progress so we won't have to discontinue him." Sally begins to protest but finds herself in a minority. She is appalled that her colleagues would consider outright lying. Finally she blurts out, "I can't believe what you are saying! This is just plain *wrong*—you are talking about lying on the evaluation form." Still she feels as if she is being swept along by a flood in which her personal beliefs and convictions will be drowned in the group's decision.

Generally speaking, laws and policies regarding this type of situation maintain that it is wrong to intend to do something that is wrong. Period. Being in a situation in which there is wrongdoing may be inevitable at times, however, when you are not in complete control. Furthermore, sometimes opportunities for achieving a good end and avoiding other greater wrongdoing can depend on cooperating with wrongdoing in some fashion. A common way to think about the justification for cooperation with wrongdoing is embodied in the principle of *material cooperation*.

The Principle of Material Cooperation

The following guidelines are offered in this principle:

- Cooperation with wrongdoing cannot be directly intended. The cooperation can be only *indirectly* not *directly* intended, perhaps occasioned solely by one's position as a member of a group.

- The more remote the cooperation, the better.
- Cooperation under these circumstances is easier to justify if the wrongdoing would happen with or without one's personal cooperation.
- The benefit that is attained by the cooperation must greatly outweigh the wrongdoing that will result.
- Finally, even appearances can support wrongdoing.

In a specific situation this general set of guidelines for when one might be able to justify cooperating with wrongdoing has to be submitted to further interpretation. Please take a few moments to look at these guidelines and try to ascertain whether you think Sally's unwilling cooperation with the group in their decision to lie about Mr. Harvey's status and progress could be justified. Jot down your thoughts about it here:

_____

_____

_____

_____

You can see that in the principle of material cooperation much hinges on the person's intent to do wrong. In the eyes of the law, actually going ahead and completing the action is a key consideration. In Sally's case, the more she tried to seek other alternatives and to persuade the others not to engage in outright lying, the more justified she would be if the group report was put forward without her being successful in changing their minds. She may decide, however, that her loyalty to her colleagues and coworkers is not sufficient excuse for her to remain silent, and she may decide to write a minority report or go public with the fact of their wrongdoing. In Chapter 8 you will be introduced to the issues of loyalty and reporting others' wrongdoing in more detail.

Protection Through Laws and Policies

As you think about living with the dictates of your conscience, keep in mind the following general resources available to professionals through laws and policies.

State Interests

Common law, the unwritten law that comes into practice over time through the lived life of a community, dictates that there is a *state interest* (i.e., responsibility) in intervening on behalf of any person under four circumstances: (1) to save your life, (2) to prevent your suicide, (3) to protect you as an innocent third party, and curiously (4) to protect you as a bearer of the "integrity of the professions." This final cause for state intervention on your behalf has evolved because of circumstances in which health professionals have been faced with requests by patients, or dictated to by policies, to act in ways that are believed by a court to be contrary to the true function of a health professional. This protection must be appealed to on a case-by-case basis.

State Licensing Laws

Professionals become certified, registered, or licensed to practice within a particular state or jurisdiction following the completion of all formal professional preparation requirements. Written into the laws governing your practice are both responsibilities and protections or rights. Among the rights is your right to practice within the dictates of your convictions. This right is weighed against the "reasonable expectations" of patients or clients who come to you for professional help.

Moral Repugnance

Moral repugnance came into the health professions' practice with the Supreme Court decision *Roe v. Wade*, which made abortion a legal right. It is a conscience clause that allows persons who believe it is morally wrong to participate in abortion procedures to be exempt from having to do so. An important aspect of this provision is that the *procedure itself* is key to whether this exemption will be upheld. It is not a protection against, say, the refusal to treat patients whose lifestyles are morally repugnant to you. Therefore it is a limited but important protection. Many have argued that a request for health professionals to assist in the lethal procedures leading to capital punishment or, should it become law, direct euthanasia would also fall under this protection. This conscience clause operates as a conscientious objection analagous to conscientious objection in war.

Institutional Policy

Finally, the *policies* of hospitals, health systems, and other health care entities may preclude your ever having to participate in processes, procedures, or other activities that are likely to run counter to the dictates of your conscience. It is always a good idea before accepting a position to be well informed of the job requirements outlined in policies. For instance, Sally may want to talk directly with Mr. Harvey about her decision and place the responsibility for discontinuing his treatment on the health plan in which she works (and which has determined the limits of his interventions). The so-called gag clauses preventing her from doing so have sometimes created moral challenges for professionals who have signed contracts agreeing not to say anything derogatory about their employer. Because of society's sensitivity to the importance of truthfulness within the health professional and patient relationship, the gag clause condition has been the subject of recent debate and legislation in Congress, the goal of many groups being to eliminate it from employment contracts.

Limits of Protection

In summary, society and many institutions that deliver high-quality health care are aware of the need for personal protection in some hopefully rare circumstances in which you feel compromised. The burden of proof regarding why you refuse to participate will fall on you, but you may be able to find support for your position in one of the above-mentioned mechanisms that have been developed. Fortunately, most health professionals are seldom in a position where they experience the deep, troubling tension of being in a situation they believe will compromise their own convictions.

SUMMARY

This chapter is but the beginning of a lifelong journey. You have chosen a career path that will require complex (and at times perplexing) moral judgments regarding patient care, health policy, and other aspects of professional life. Many such judgments will have significance in terms of your own moral life, that of your profession, and of society. But the path is not one that you must forge anew every step of the way. This chapter introduces you to some basic ways of thinking about the sources of morality on which you will draw, the general relevance of ethics to your everyday professional life, and the personal protections you can expect if you are faced with potential compromises of your convictions. As you study the next chapters you will be better able to appreciate the contribution of these basic considerations.

Questions for Thought and Discussion

1. Imagine a situation that may arise in your professional career that would pose a challenge to your personal morality. What about this situation creates the challenge?

_____

_____

_____

2. Using the code of ethics from your own chosen profession, identify three or four basic moral guidelines that you will be expected to follow.

_____

_____

_____

3. Search in your newspaper for an article about health care involving ethical issues.

   a. What are the main issues?

     _____

     _____

     _____

   b. What types of decisions will have to be made (or have been made) about the right or wrong thing to do in this instance?

     _____

     _____

     _____

References

1. Sim, J., Purtilo, R. 1991. An ethical analysis of the duty to treat persons who have AIDS: Homosexual patients as a test case. *Physical Therapy* 71(9):650–656.
2. Hume, D. 1996. *An Inquiry Concerning the Principles of Morals* (2nd ed.). La Salle, IL: Open Court.

2

All You Need to Know about Ethics Approaches and Theories—I: Background Information and Case-Driven Approaches

Objectives

The student should be able to:
- Describe the significance of several basic distinctions between ethical theories and approaches: deductive versus inductive, theories of action versus theories of virtue, individualistic versus common good theories, reason versus emotion-based theories.
- Name two roles that emotion plays in ethical reflection.
- Distinguish metaethics from normative ethics.
- Distinguish between absolutist and relativist ethical theories and approaches.
- Name five types of normative ethical theories and approaches.
- Describe a narrative and what it means to take a narrative approach to an ethical issue or problem.
- Describe the contribution that Gilligan and others who stress relationship have made to our understanding of morality.
- Discuss several contributions that feminist and postmodernist approaches have made to our understanding of ethical issues and problems.
- Describe how the idea of care is used in professional ethics and what its function is in the health professional and patient relationship.
- Compare casuistry with other inductive approaches.

New Terms and Ideas You Will Encounter in This Chapter

Theories (and approaches)
Deductive

Inductive
Theories of action

Virtue theories
Individualistic approaches
Common good theories
   Aggregate
   Communitarian
Role of reason
Role of emotions
Metaethics
Absolutism
Relativism

Normative theories
Deontology
Teleology
Case-driven approaches
Narrative approaches
Feminist approaches
Postmodernism
Ethics of care
Casuistry

Topics in This Chapter Introduced in an Earlier Chapter

Topic	Introduced In	Discussed In This Chapter On
Three uses of ethics in everyday life	Chapter 1	Pages 14 and 15
The story of Mr. and Mrs. Harvey	Chapter 1	Page 4

Introduction

In this chapter and the next you will be introduced to the most general level of ethical reflection, that which is presented in ethical theories and approaches. A complete *theory* is a general overview or statement that begins with an assumption about the very nature of doing right and wrongdoing, of virtuous or vicious character, and includes how humans can go about achieving one and avoiding the other. In contrast an *approach* does not propose to be a complete system or model but to be an aid to existing theories or other approaches.

Ethical theories and approaches are tools to help organize your beliefs about human existence, especially in regard to your beliefs about how the world operates in relation to human freedom and responsibility, how society really functions best, and how human relationships are sustained and nurtured. In Chapter 1 I suggested three general ways that ethics has usefulness in your everyday life. If you remember these, jot them down here:

1. _____

2. _____

3. _____

In case you have forgotten, the three ways are (1) to analyze moral issues and problems, (2) to help resolve conflicts among morals, and (3) to move toward action when faced with an ethical issue or problem. (If you want to review them in more detail, return to Chapter 1, pages 14 and 15).

In this and the next three chapters you will become better equipped to travel from ethical theories or approaches to actual assessment and especially to resolution of a specific issue or problem. First you have an opportunity to learn some important background information about how to become fluent in the language and logic of ethics and what the two basic levels of ethics are.

BECOMING A PART OF THE ETHICS CONVERSATION

Your familiarity with several basic distinctions that divide ethical theories and approaches will allow you to become a part of the ethics conversation because you will be able to identify where a writer or other person is coming from in an ethics discussion or debate. Once you have identified your own or another's thinking you will be able to enter into the ethical discussion more confidently.

Deductive and Inductive Theories and Approaches

Deductive theories and approaches propose that the human mind (usually the faculty of reason) is capable of discerning truths about the moral life from a pattern of visible laws in the universe or from some set of general rules or principles that can be discerned by humans through intuition, revelation, or other reliable means. The general truths become a basis to guide action in concrete situations.

Inductive theories and approaches start with concrete experience. Some suggest that these theories and approaches are less a system for guidance and more a rejection of the belief that reliable action-guides can be found, the least likely being those found in places where deductive theorists turn.

Between these two extremes are many theories that give credence to some combination of human rationality (or other intellectual resource): One is the dialectic approach, which proposes an interplay between abstract action-guides and concrete situations; another is a casuistical approach (discussed later in this chapter), which depends heavily on everyday situations that are related by common ethical themes.

To Do or To Be?

Another type of tension has existed through the ages. Ethicists have debated over the question, Does the moral life fundamentally demand of you to do certain right things and avoid other wrong ones? Or, at the basis of morality is there a mandate to *be* a certain kind of person (i.e., a person of virtue)?

Theories of the former sort are classified as *theories of action*, while those emphasizing character trait formation are *virtue theories*. Perhaps the correct answer lies in discovering the appropriate *relationship* between action and virtue, although exactly which ultimately takes precedence in the moral life is open to discussion. You will learn more about both sides of this debate in later discussions in this chapter as well as in Chapter 3.

Individuals or Communities as Units of Concern?

In recent years there has been renewed inquiry regarding the appropriate moral relationship of individuals to the larger community in which they live. Should individual or community well-being be the standard? This is important for many reasons, the most obvious being that the answer to that query will guide ethical practices and policies about right and wrong actions as well as form the basis for deciding which virtues should be applauded or negatively sanctioned. *Individualistic* ethical theories and approaches take individual well-being as the standard by which to make correct moral judgments. The individual as the focus of concern is a recent phenomenon in the history of ideas. Protection of individual rights and a focus on individual autonomy and happiness are important goals in this approach: This position is seen in many aspects of modern health care. For example, informed consent is one safeguard for individuals. At the same time, some ethicists are joining others in wondering if modern Western societies have gone awry in placing individual well-being at the highest pinnacle of society's values and duties (i.e., its morality).

In *common good* theories and approaches the community as a whole is the common denominator of concern. Their strength is their attention to the deep (essential) interdependence among humans. They help to set checks and balances on individual self-interest. These theorists focus on communal arrangements that they believe assure the larger society and its subgroups will survive and flourish. As you might expect, fairness in the distribution of scarce resources and a deep respect for the environment and other resources that sustain human health are an important (though by no means the only) focus of such theories and approaches.

Attempts to strike a reasonable balance between the extremes of these two positions have been made: *Aggregate* approaches propose that the major criterion for an acceptable moral community is that each and every individual realizes her or his own basic values and upholds her or his own duties. *Communitarian* approaches depend on reaching agreements (e.g., social contracts, consensus building, utilitarian weighing of benefits and burdens) that are acceptable to all. Both aggregate and communitarian approaches caution that unbridled expressions of individual rights cannot be tolerated.

Reason or Emotion for Reliable Moral Judgment?

Deductivists maintain that your faculty of *reason* is your internal website where you can go and search to find the appropriate ingredients for ethical assessment, movement toward resolution of problems, and action. Of course, different theories and approaches might assert that your reason is informed through direct revelation by God or through intuition or natural laws, but rationalists agree that your faculty of reason finally does the essential work of ethical reflection.

This approach has led to considerable debate about the significance of *emotion* in ethical reflection. Strict rationalists view emotion as too subjective and unpredictable to serve as a reliable guide.

At the same time, there are convincing arguments for assigning emotion at least two roles in ethical reflection. First, there is the fact that when you encounter a morally perplexing situation you *feel* discomfort, anxiety, anger, or some other disturbing emotion. Emotion is an "alert" system. Recall Chapter 1 when Sally Lim became angry and confused because she realized her colleagues were preparing to tell a lie about Mr. Harvey's progress. Emotion was the painful warning signal that she had "stubbed her toe" on her moral journey through life. Nancy Sherman, a contemporary philosopher working on the place of emotion in morality, proposes that emotions are "modes of sensitivity that record what is morally salient and . . . communicate those concerns to self and others."[1] Your emotions grab your attention. A second role for emotion emerges: it assists you in deciding whom to help and when and where. In this regard, emotions also are motivators: sometimes it is an emotional response to wrongdoing, tragedy, or a heroic act that stirs a person out of lethargy and into action on someone else's behalf. In short, ethical reflection without the life infused into it by emotional responses to specific situations could be vacuous and misleading.

Despite the caveats traditionally posed by rationalists, many ethicists today acknowledge a positive role for emotion in ethical reflection: it alerts, focuses attention, communicates where the real problems lie, motivates, and increases one's knowledge about complex situations.

Summary

In summary, several on-going points of difference distinguish ethical theories and approaches from each other. Not all theories or approaches address all these questions. To be "in the know" you would be well advised to watch for signs that would place a particular approach or theory within one or more of the preceding distinctions.

PARTS OF ETHICAL STUDY

Before going to an examination of specific approaches and theories it will be useful for your future work in ethics to become acquainted with the two basic levels of discourse in ethics: metaethics and normative ethics. Almost all the ethical reflection you do relevant to everyday life problems is in the area of normative ethics, so several normative approaches and theories are described in more detail in the last discussions of this chapter and in Chapter 3.

Metaethics

Metaethics tries to discover the nature and meaning of ethical reasons we propose as valid for making judgments about morality. How do we know if there are ultimate truths about morality? Does the certainty come from our lived experience? From revelation or scripture? From reasoning? Is there a "natural law" from which humans can discern truths about right or wrong? These are just some questions metaethics deals with. You will recognize some of them as belonging to deductive or inductive schools of thought. An understanding of metaethics requires that you become more aware of your beliefs—religious, philosophical, what you have been taught or told—and how you imagine them to influence what is right or wrong. In Chapter 1 you wrote down some of your own ideas about the sources that inform your thinking. In doing so, you were doing important work related to metaethics because the sources of your moral belief are the starting point from which your own thinking and action will be justified. Of course, over time, you may modify any of these aspects of moral understanding.

An Example of Metaethical Approaches: Absolutism and Relativism

Let us return to the Harveys' story in Chapter 1 for just a minute. Surely you have some idea of what you think ought to be done regarding the predicament Mr. Harvey and his caregivers are facing. When you first read their story did you feel certain from the beginning that you knew *why* a particular course of action should be taken? Did you wonder why anyone would ever worry about the alternatives because it was so obvious? Did you think, There is a good (moral) reason why everyone should always do such and such? Yes _____ No _____

If you answered yes to these questions *and* if your reflection is based on believing that there are clear, unchanging reasons for always taking your course of action, then you were thinking as an absolutist. *Absolutist metaethical theories* rest on the notion that what is right is based on knowledge that can be known to be a truth. In your consideration of sources of morality, some of you probably stated your religious beliefs as one important source. Religious truths are believed to be absolute, truths that can be known to be truths because they are from a divine source, usually recorded in scripture. Other theories add that truths may become evident through the working of natural forces (natural law theory) or by intuition. Even in these theories, however, there may be differences of opinion about the exact way that these truths provide guidance for everyday decisions. Some (e.g., fundamentalists) argue that there is knowledge from the source to the direct application of any decision. Others (e.g., deductive rationalists) would counter that the faculty of human reason must intervene to discern right or wrong in any given situation, interpreting what the absolute truth requires at any specific moment.

Perhaps you answered no to the above question. You are quite sure that there are no true reasons to guide what is right or wrong or that if there are such reasons, you could not be sure of ascertaining them: One person's (or group's) morally right judgment is another's wrong. If this is your approach, you are reasoning as a relativist.

Relativistic metaethical theories rest on the assumption that ethical statements are not known to be ultimately true or false. In the end, what any society, group, or individual believes is right can be as legitimately defended as what another society, group, or individual asserts. All is relative, although many different groups may agree regarding the course of action that should be taken. Postmodernist thinkers are one group holding such a position. You will encounter more about their position later in this chapter. Basically they suggest that the richness of our plurality as humans goes to the very root of our makeup and that ultimate truths are conjectures by groups to try to gain power or control over others.

Do you think you are basically an absolutist or a relativist?

Absolutist _____ Relativist _____ Why?_____

This example of metaethical considerations should illustrate that your acquaintance with the metaethics level of ethical theory is relevant in several ways: first, it is important for you to be aware of the lines of thinking by which you yourself believe that judgments of right and wrong can be made with certainty—or perhaps, never can be made with certainty; second, in disagreements with professional peers, patients, and others about important moral positions, often it is critical to be able to figure out the basis of their justification for their positions for you to know whether you can hope for more consensus. It is difficult to persuade someone to change his mind if God has spoken directly to that person through revelation or scripture. Finally, as an educated person you should have the capability to listen knowledgeably at all levels of ethical reflection in everyday discourse about important moral issues and problems in society.

For our present purposes this brief discussion of metaethical considerations provides you with an adequate working knowledge of the role such theories play in overall ethical thought. In your lifelong learning you may wish or need to know more about metaethical theories. Most basic ethics textbooks have a section on metaethics or, as it is sometimes called, critical ethics.

Normative Ethics

Normative ethics asks more concrete questions related to morality. What types of acts are morally right or wrong? What are the morally praiseworthy or blameworthy traits (virtues) of individuals or institutions? What values are morally good or bad for the harmonious functioning of society and the welfare of individuals?

No matter what position you take in regard to the distinctions between theories and approaches discussed in the first section of this chapter and no matter which normative theory you use, the encounter with a real situation involving a patient, colleague, other people, a rule, a policy, or a practice is what will motivate you to engage in ethical reflection. Therefore you will be better able to grasp the importance and role of normative ethics by beginning your inquiry with a real situation. I have chosen the situation of Ronald Rachels, someone I spoke with when he called me to discuss a quandary he was in about what he should do. He gave me permission to share this story with you because we agreed it raises moral themes you will encounter time and time again, even if you never meet this *exact* situation:

THE STORY OF RONALD RACHELS

A radiologic technologist, whom we will call Ronald Rachels, works in a large community hospital. He is responsible for performing many radiologic procedures each day and takes his job seriously. Patients who arrive at his department quickly learn that Ron is a bright spot in their otherwise anxiety-producing ordeal of having x-rays or imaging. He explains everything to the patients in language they can understand and tries to make them comfortable while waiting and during their procedures. If there are necessary delays, he explains why.

Two weeks ago, Ron had an experience that upset him, and he's not sure what to do about it: A young woman, whom we will call Pamela Faden, had met Ron while her x-rays were taken before her first surgery for abdominal cancer. This day she came back. She remembered Ron and greeted him. He learned that this 23-year-old woman had had a difficult time following abdominal surgery and had not been able to leave the hospital. X-rays were ordered to try to discern the cause of her ongoing problem.

The x-rays were developed. He happened to walk by the radiology resident who was reading the printouts and was astonished to see a large scalpel in her abdominal cavity, lodged near her liver. The resident instructed Ron to take several additional pictures, not explaining why, though Ron of course knew. The patient said, "Did you find something? Why are you taking so many x-rays?"

"We just want to be sure we have all the views," he replied nervously. She said with anxiety, "Is anything wrong?"

"That's what the x-rays may help to tell us," he answered.

After all the x-rays had been developed, he heard the resident talking on the telephone to Dr. Kristansen, who performed the surgery. A few minutes later Dr. Kristansen arrived. When he saw the scalpel he turned ashen and muttered, "This is *not* good, *not* good." He gathered up the x-rays and hurried out of the room.

Ron wanted to say, "Are you going to tell her?" but he didn't. He knew Dr.

Kristansen was on his way to see the patient and also was afraid the doctor may have been insulted by such a question.

Today Ron is transferring a portable x-ray unit to another part of the hospital when he sees Pamela Faden in the elevator. She says, "Well, they didn't find anything on those x-rays."

"Did the physician talk with you about them?" Ron asks, feeling tense.

"No—he hasn't said anything at all."

"Well," Ron says, "You have the right to know the results if you want to."

She immediately looks concerned. He wants to say something to reassure her, but the words fail him.

The elevator door opens, and Ron says a hurried good-bye. He feels a gnawing in the pit of his stomach, but he can't immediately figure out what, if anything, he should do next.

It is not surprising that Ron Rachels is distressed because something definitely is wrong. In fact, we might wonder about a health professional who felt no emotion at all about this situation: A young woman with cancer is suffering; a scalpel has been left in her abdomen; communication between her and her physician has broken down. Maybe, he, Ron, has said too much—or too little—to help this patient and physician, both of whom have had some bad news to confront. He is not sure how far he should go in revealing directly to the patient what he knows.

This story provides you with an opportunity to see the role various ethical normative approaches and theories may play when you are trying to analyze what the real problem is, when you are moving to resolve ethical problems, and finally, when it is time for you to act.

Five useful approaches and theories you may pick and choose from in ethical reflection are the focus of the rest of this chapter and the next:

1. Story- or case-driven approaches; all of these fall within the inductive method.
2. Casuistry, which looks for more general ethics themes among stories or cases.
3. Deontological theories.
4. Teleological theories.

These latter two mouthfuls can be broken down into more digestible pieces by looking at their roots. The root word "deonto" means duty. The root word "telos" means end. Already you can see a distinction developing. Deontological theories rely on duties (actually duties, rights, or other forms of action), whereas teleological ones rely on ends or consequences to determine when one is acting rightly or wrongly. Deonto are *means* theories; teleo are *ends* theories.

5. Virtue theories.

CASE-DRIVEN APPROACHES: THE STORY ITSELF IS CENTRAL

Among the inductive approaches to ethics, all hold that morally relevant information about the situation is embedded in the story itself. Some claim that you need not or will not be able to appeal to any other source for further insight during your ethical reflection; others view the content and organization of the story as being the key, but not the exclusive, source of ethical assessment and decision making. Whether you think that ethical reflection relies entirely on "knowing" the story is something you will be better able to conclude when you have finished surveying all the approaches presented in this chapter and Chapter 3.

Narrative Approaches

Narrative approaches rely on the story, based on the observation that humans pass on information, impute and explore meaning in their and others' lives, commemorate and celebrate, denounce, clarify, get affirmation, and, overall, become a part of a community through the hearing and telling of stories. These stories are passed down from generation to generation among families or whole communities. Sometimes stories have been fictionalized in novels, poems, plays, songs, or other literary forms. "Narrative" is the technical term applied to the story's characters, events, and ordering of events (e.g., the plot), although in health care ethics and legal circles you will more often see the term "case."[2] Since morality is about human narratives of individuals and communities, narrative ethicists conclude that moral judgment about doing the right thing and becoming a virtuous person must rely on the analysis and understanding of narratives. Kathyrn Hunter, a contemporary leader in narrative approaches to ethics within health care, reiterates this point, noting that through narratives

> [W]e spin and untangle explanatory accounts of the way the world works and how we and our fellow human beings act in every conceivable circumstance. Memories of the past and ideas of the future are expressed in narrative accounts of how the world was and how it will, or *should*, become.[3] [italics mine]

Her emphasis on "should" underscores the narrative ethicists' position that future choices of individuals and communities rightfully are shaped through understanding and taking seriously the information and lessons embedded in narrative accounts.

Ron Rachels' situation is revealed to you as a narrative. One thing probably disturbing to him is the fragmented narrative he himself has received. He lacks certain information about the patient, the physician, and their exchanges that he needs to be confident of the morality of the situation. This means that he not only is without facts and details but also may feel he lacks the information to make a valid judgment about the real significance and meaning of the events unfolding before him. There are no principles or other external sources of information that are going to fill in those blanks. In that regard the morality is indeed ensconced in the story.

What are some of the questions *you* have about Ron's situation? Are there some facts missing? Some standards, policies, accepted procedures you would want to know to judge the situation? If so, jot them down here:

_____

_____

_____

The desire to fill in the blanks in your knowledge of the situation helps you to see the importance of the narrative for correct interpretations of the situation and, consequently, valid moral judgments.

Ron's narrative also highlights that in complex situations there is not just one but several narrative accounts. Suppose this story was titled The Story of Dr. Kristansen. What different concerns might Dr. Kristansen express regarding his role, his relationships with the patient Pam Faden and with Ron, or anything else? It would be a different story than the one I described from my discussion with this young health professional. (Did you guess he was young? How?) Or suppose this story was titled The Story of Pam Faden. Surely this young patient's account would include details about her life and experience, her response to her illness, and her hopes, dreams, and fears. These details would alter inexorably what Ron's story taken alone conveys. Narrative ethics approaches require diligent efforts to consider as many perspectives of the situation as possible before interpreting the situation for its moral significance.

Hunter further elucidates the role of narrative approaches by comparing moral reasoning to clinical reasoning. Clinical reasoning requires that you be able to gather relevant information and correctly apply your clinical knowledge and skills in a way that will meet your desired goal of good patient care. To do this well you will have to be attentive to the details of each patient's unique history and present situation. Likewise, moral reasoning requires that you be able to gather relevant information and correctly apply your ethical knowledge and skills in the process of ethical reflection. This too requires great attention to the details of each narrative.[4]

As you continue to explore approaches and theories for dealing with complex ethical issues and problems, this brief introduction to narrative approaches will serve as a reminder of the strengths that this approach can bring to ethical reflection during your professional practice.

Approaches Emphasizing Relationship

Some case-driven ethical approaches search for the central moral themes of a story in an examination of the human relationships revealed in the story. Ethical issues or problems are embedded in the relationships. Therefore ethical reflection requires searching for what will make this human relationship (or relationships) thrive or perish. In Chapter 1 you learned that morality describes the practices that allow humans to live together peacefully and harmoniously, that is, *in community*. An emphasis on relationships makes sense, psychologically speaking, since the quality of human relationships will indeed determine whether humans in communities will tend to thrive or languish.

Not surprisingly, this approach has been promoted and refined by psychologists, particularly those working in the area of moral development. Others, particularly feminist ethicists and other postmodernist thinkers, have added new and important dimensions to the discussion of relationship.

Carol Gilligan Introduces In a Different Voice

Gilligan is an important leader in this arena, her work having been drawn from a widely accepted model of children's moral development advanced by Harvard psychologist Lawrence Kohlberg. He hypothesized that children go through stages of moral development similar to cognitive development and that children become more independent and autonomous as they mature as moral beings. His work became a—if not the—dominant moral development theory in the early 1980s.[5] At that time, Gilligan, then a graduate student, noted that Kohlberg's work depended on studies of boys and young men. She repeated some of the work with girls and young women, only to discover that her subjects conceptualized ethical issues and problems differently than their male counterparts. This led to the publication of *In a Different Voice: Psychological Theory and Women's Development*, detailing her findings that girls had a high sensitivity to how various actions would affect their important relationships (i.e., with parents, friends, teachers, or other authority figures).[6] She concluded that girls' "awareness of the connection between people gives rise to a recognition of responsibility for another.[7]" Furthermore, her subjects did not see moral maturity as being characterized by an increasing *independence* from everyone else, rather by decisions that would result in *deeper and more effective connections* and relationships to significant others and the larger community. Her findings made it obvious that attention to relationship and how relationship is nourished was important to at least half the human race as they struggled to become moral beings!

Further Research

This work became one vital basis for thinkers in other disciplines besides psychology to affirm that relationship figures into morality.[8,9] Ethicists who had been emphasizing this dimension became more active in refining their understanding of the ways relationship is central.[10–12] (Several of their contributions are discussed in this chapter and the next.) Moreover, further examination showed that while girls and women may be socialized to think in terms of sustaining relationship, the significance of Gilligan's findings are by no means gender specific.[13] For example, Ron Rachels' reflection on his situation suggests that he believes his relationship with Pam Faden has several significant dimensions. Can you name some of them?

_____

_____

_____

_____

You might have listed that he is aware he has significant power to determine what will happen in Pam Faden's situation because of the nature of his professional expertise, his access to the x-rays and to Dr. Kristansen himself, and also because of his secret regarding the likely source of her abdominal discomfort. Or you might have noted that he is aware that the type of "connection" they have might place some responsibility on him to tell her what he knows. He detects that she trusts him as well as Dr. Kristansen. Perhaps he wonders if her trust has any relevance in determining what he should do.

In summary, proponents of a relationship approach to stories maintain that Ron's search for and grasp of the significance of the relationship holds the key to his ability to resolve the conflict he is experiencing.

Feminist Ethics and Postmodernism: All Those Voices and the Social Context Besides

Partially because her findings initially were assumed to highlight gender-specific differences, the decade following the publication of Gilligan's *In a Different Voice* led to considerable growth in publications by feminists and others who were engaged in feminist and postmodernist examinations of ethics.* *Feminist approaches and theories* analyze stories or cases to make careful critiques of prevailing ethical theories, approaches, and methods, exposing their relevance (or lack of it) for women's experience.[14,15] They also joined feminists in other disciplines who were, and continue to be, committed to showing how social practices and institutional structures are important aspects of the spoken (or unspoken) narrative of women's experience and how many negatively affect women.[16–18] Some feminists are postmodernists, the latter being a group who are involved not only in critiquing but also in denying the validity of prevailing theories, approaches, and methods.

---

*For an excellent summary of various aspects of the feminist approach see Karen Lebacqz. 1995. Feminism. In Reich, W.T. (Ed.), *Encyclopedia of Bioethics* (rev. ed., vol. 2). New York: Macmillan, pp. 808–816. Her references also contain an extensive list of feminist writers.

Deep Diversity as a Factor

Postmodernists assert that since there are *radical* differences among peoples and cultures, no one set of moral rules or values is a valid guide "across the board" or even "across a relationship."[19] This position flies in the face of traditional ethics approaches, as you will see in Chapter 3. The postmodernist approach is like other inductive approaches because the specific experiences each party brings to that time and place (i.e., to the story) is all you have for understanding what should be done. However postmodernists assert more: for persons of one social class, racial group, ethnic community, or gender to pretend to understand the situation of persons in another is viewed by the postmodernist as being an expression of social elitism, racism, ethnocentrism, or sexism. To illustrate the narrowness of our own perspectives, please think with me for a moment about how quickly our understanding of other people reaches a limit.

Try to think about the characteristics of age, physical appearance, race, social class, gender, type of job or career, sexual preference, religion, or other details that would be likely to give a person a position of authority

- in your class
- in a small Midwestern town dominated by German Lutheran immigrants
- in an affluent suburb of Los Angeles
- in Spanish Harlem
- in Tokyo
- in a Hmong village of Cambodia
- in a farming community in Nepal
- in a monastery on Mount Athos

Our provincialism quickly hems in our ability to make wise judgments about how communities are conceived and operate peacefully and harmoniously. This leads postmodernists to assert that we underestimate how deep the diversity of human value and understanding of duty (i.e., morality) goes, and so we simply impose our own morality, to our own advantage. One important contribution, then, of postmodernist thinking to ethical reflection is its urgent call for attention to diversity.

Institutional Arrangements as a Factor

Above I mentioned that feminists study the influence of institutional and other social arrangements on the well-being of women. Postmodernists emphasize how the larger social and institutional arrangements of a society influence individual action and relationships in general. Ethical reflection requires recognition of the powerful influence of each player's (and some groups') "place" in society.

In health care, your recognition of imbalances of power among individuals because of the types of institutions and other social arrangements society condones will be a key factor in your ability to interpret complex situations accurately.* If you noted the difference in power between Ron Rachels and Pam Faden or between Ron Rachels and the physician Kristansen, *because of their relative status and assigned roles within the institution of health care*, you were inherently attending to the social or institutional influences that postmodernists herald as relevant considerations in ethical reflection.

In summary, in story-driven, postmodernist approaches the first major task is to be not only humble in the face of rich diversity but also respectful of deep differences and, to the extent possible, to show respect for those differences in your relationships with others. The second is to take seriously the influence of the larger social context of interaction.

Care: A Silver Thread in Relationships

So far you have been introduced to ethical approaches that use individuals' and communities' stories

- to discover the moral relevance of a situation
- to highlight the moral significance of relationships in the situation
- as a means of being attentive to deep differences among humans.

You have also been warned of power differentials that arise in structures and institutions that can undermine the well-being of some persons and groups. Taken together they stress the importance of attending to the uniqueness of each individual, relationships, and the social context.

The idea of care and caring is a common theme that has woven itself among many of the above approaches to give them shape and substance. Today an approach called the *ethics of care* is being used and refined in bioethics. In an ethics of care the major questions are, What does my commitment to caring for this person require me to do? and What kind of a person must I become to best be able to express that I care?

The desire to explore these questions should not be surprising since ample opportunities to express care for others present themselves in the health professional and patient encounter. As you think about Ron Rachels' role as a health professional, what opportunities does he have to express caring toward the patient Pam Faden? toward the physician?

_____

_____

---

*For a more thorough discussion of the peculiarities of the health care environment see Ruth Purtilo and Amy Haddad: The environment of health care institutions. In *Health Professional and Patient Interaction* (5th ed.). Philadelphia: W.B. Saunders, pp. 29–48.

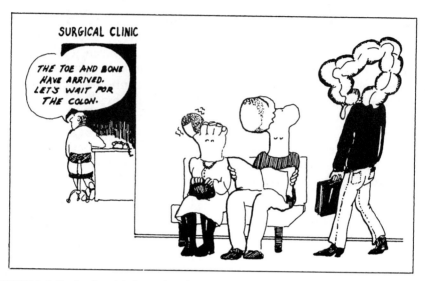

FIGURE 2–1 Professionals' view of patients.
From Purtilo, R. 1982. *Vård, Vårdare, Vårdad.* Umeå, Sweden: Esselte Studium, p. 139. (Swedish translation of Purtilo, R. 1978. *Health Professional and Patient Interaction.* Philadelphia: W.B. Saunders.)

Care is the language adopted in the health professions' ethical literature to emphasize the imperative that professionals must keep a focus on the well-being of the whole person. Although the terms "health care" and "managed care" may simply mean dealing with the patient in the technical sense, ethicists use the term with the broader common connotation of really caring about the person. It is closely related to the age-old notion of compassion, with compassion being the disposition that gives rise to caring behaviors.[20] Care requires health professionals to direct full attention to the well-being of the person.[21] This focus of attention frequently is challenged in an era of clinical specialization and high technology: Intervention is so specialized that a particular disease, symptom, body part, or biological system becomes the focus of attention.[22,23] Fear of the dehumanizing effect that a fragmented focus will have on both the health professional and patient is illustrated in Figure 2–1.

Managed "care," with its emphasis on efficiency and cost savings and its reliance on protocols that standardize treatments according to whole groups of patient *types,* also has become a basis for concern.[24] Can you think of other barriers to care? If so, list them here:

_____

_____

_____

Gilligan's work factors in modern explorations of this idea too. She identified the major difference of perspective between males and females to be that boys and men were increasingly concerned with equality or justice while girls and women were increasingly compelled by care. You have seen that the gender distinction is not radical, that rather it points to characteristics either gender may manifest but may easily be expressed by most females because of the way they have been socialized since childhood.

Nursing ethics has been an important vehicle for developing the ethics of care. As nursing ethics became more sophisticated, in the early 1980s the idea of care emerged as a central theme in studies designed to characterize the profession's identity.[25-28] Since then additional exciting work has helped to refine what caring entails. For instance, maternal activities that foster growth and conscientiousness have been one key focus[29] that have produced advocates of the position as well as critics. Advocates find deep similarities. Critics voice concern that while caring for others is an activity associated with the mother's role, women's traits often are devalued. Therefore reliance on the model of motherhood may not fully convey the complexity and importance of caring activities nurses and others engage in to respect and respond according to the dignity of patients, clients, and others.[30]

Some ethicists worry that an accent on the silver thread of care may deflect attention from injustices woven into the basic warp and woof of health care structures, placing all the responsibility to care on individual professionals in the face of policies and practices that are barriers to it. Despite these legitimate concerns, the emphasis on morality understood through the lens of care gives shape to many of the important considerations you have been introduced to in this chapter. Since an ethics of care is still developing, continue to watch for articles and other opportunities to refine your own interpretation of what care entails in the health professional and patient relationship.

APPROACH—CASUISTRY

Casuistry (kas-you-is-tree) is an approach that also is case or story dependent, but casuists hold that ultimately you can find valid common moral themes among cases. Each such set of cases creates a "paradigm case." This latter assumption distinguishes it from the approaches you have been introduced to so far, where the truth about the moral situation is embedded solely in each case or story and similarities among them are simply happenstance.

Casuistry as an approach to analyzing moral issues or problems has its roots in medieval times. Recently it has been modernized by two eminent leaders in the fields of bioethics and philosophy, Albert Jonsen and Steven Toulmin.[31] They have shown that casuistry relies on a formal and systematic method of closely examining cases. The first step is to identify the part of the story that caught your attention. What makes you think there might be a moral issue or moral problem? In the story of Ron Rachels, Pamela Faden, and the physician Kristansen it might be "competent patients have a right to know what is happening in regard to their own health and medical care, and Pamela Faden is being kept in the dark," or "health professionals have a responsibility to be truthful," and Dr. Kristansen is not telling Pamela what is going on. At this step it is also necessary to identify the specific circumstances of the story (i.e., the "facts") that were the most important in leading you to decide what the moral issues are. You can name them:

_____

_____

Some I would emphasize are the presence of the scalpel, the apparent lack of communication with Pamela, her serious illness, her anxiety about what is happening, and Ron Rachels' own anxiety and frustration. Are these similar to what you named? In Chapter 5 you will be introduced to several categories of facts that are almost always relevant to your decision making in situations that present moral issues or problems. That will give you more confidence that you really have found out as much as you can about a situation.

Casuists then compare this type of case with other stories that share common *themes*. I would say the Ron Rachels' situation has the themes of truth telling, trust, professional duty or responsibility to relieve suffering, and patient choice, to name some. These themes also are present in, say, the story of the Harveys (Chapter 1), so the two stories are similar in some important areas.

Finally, analogies between the two cases are highlighted, but significant differences are identified. In this process the casuist would argue that you should be able to discern the true peculiarities of Ron Rachels' situation and what you ought to do. In this, as in the other approaches in this chapter, the story itself is the resource for discerning what should be done.

SUMMARY

In the approaches in this chapter the narrative, story, or case holds the key to the knowledge you need for doing the right thing or exercising appropriate character traits in the situation conveyed in the story. My goal has been to show you their strengths and how they contribute to the richness of ethical thought and action in the health care world you are entering. In Chapter 3 you will be introduced (or, for some of you, reintroduced) to ethical approaches bioethicists have more commonly relied on to analyze moral issues and problems. Generally speaking, the latter approaches and theories find no fault with the fact-finding dimensions of the case-driven approaches.

The departure comes at the point of discerning the resources necessary for you to decide the right thing to do or what makes a good person or institution. In the more traditional approaches you are encouraged to use but also look beyond the story for guidance—in the form of maxims, potential consequences, principles, or dispositions.

Questions for Thought and Discussion

1. This is an opportunity for the class to create a narrative of a patient, Esther Korn. It is a group exercise about a health care situation that came to the attention of the hospital ethics committee. The whole class can participate in the discussion as members of the ethics committee, and five people will assume various important roles.

    The ethics committee has been asked to give advice on whether Esther Korn should be sent back home or to a nursing home.

    > Esther Korn, a 27-year-old woman, has been admitted to the hospital with a diagnosis of dehydration and serious bruises from a fall sustained in her home. She was found by a neighbor, Anna Knight, who says she stops by Esther's home daily because Ms. Korn has lived alone with her eight cats since being discharged from a state mental institution with a diagnosis of involutional paranoia, which is believed to be under control with medications. From the degree of dehydration the health professionals believe that Ms. Korn was very dehydrated before she fell and that she had been lying on the floor for at least a day. The emergency medical team who brought her to the hospital described her home as "filthy, full of dirty dishes and clothes strung all over, with cat droppings everywhere."
    >
    > Now, five days later, Ms. Korn seems confused about where she is but does know her own name. She says, over and over, "Let me out of here! I want to go home!" Her sister, whom she has not seen "for years" (according to Anna Knight), has a telephone message service and does not return the nurses' calls. The nurses are not in complete agreement, but most of the staff believe Esther would be better off in an institution for her own safety. Anna Knight and the local priest, who visits her regularly, also have strong opinions about where she would be better off.

    Five people will be "story tellers" to provide some missing parts to her story: one will be Esther, the other four will be significant others in her life. Together the class can create a profile that will give much more information about who she is and what may, in fact, be in her best interests in this difficult question facing the ethics committee:

    Person A   Write a few paragraphs about Esther from Anna's perspective and what Anna thinks should be done.

Person B Write about her story from the priest's perspective and what he would recommend.

Person C Write about her from her long-lost-sister's perspective and what she would recommend.

Person D Write a report from the point of view of the primary nurse and what she thinks.

Person E Speak as Esther, giving some background, what kind of person she believes herself to be, what is important to her, and so on.

When each of the five story tellers has completed this part of the exercise, read the notes aloud to the ethics committee (i.e., rest of the group). After everyone has heard the "bigger picture":

- What should be done?
- What influences your thinking the most?
- Which values do you think are the most prominent in this discussion?
- Did anything that was said in these stories change your mind about your initial thoughts regarding what should be done? If so, explain.
- Discuss what the health professionals must do to show *caring* in their relationship with Esther Korn.

2. Find a news story in your local newspaper that alleges unethical or illegal behavior by a person or group. Make a list of the "facts" about them that are included in the story. Now make a list of the "unanswered questions" (e.g., person's life, possible motives, personality, lifestyle and needs, influences). With this enriched picture, what kinds of moral judgments might you better be able to make about him, her, or them?

References

1. Sherman, N. 1995. Emotions. In Reich, W.T. (Ed.), *Encyclopedia of Bioethics* (rev. ed., vol. 2). New York: Macmillan, pp. 64–70. Citation page 65.
2. Hunter, K. 1995. Narrative. In Reich, W.T. (Ed.), *Encyclopedia of Bioethics* (rev. ed., vol. 4). New York: Macmillan, p. 1789.
3. Ibid., p. 1790.
4. Ibid., p. 1791.
5. Kohlberg, L. 1981. *The Philosophy of Moral Development: Moral Stages and the Idea of Justice*. San Francisco: Harper and Row.
6. Gilligan, C. 1982. *In a Different Voice—Psychological Theory and Women's Development*. Cambridge, MA: Harvard University Press.
7. Ibid., p. 30.
8. Jecker, N. 1993. Impartiality and special relations. In Meyers, D.T., Kipnis, K.,

Murphy, C., Jr. (Eds.), *Kindred Matters: Rethinking the Philosophy of the Family.* Ithaca, NY: Cornell University Press, pp. 41–58.

9. Benhabib, S. 1987. The generalized and the concrete other: The Kohlberg-Gilligan controversy and moral theory. In Kittay, E.F., Meyers, D.T. (Eds.), *Women and Moral Theory.* Lanham, MD: Rowman and Littlefield, pp. 154–177.

10. May, W.F. 1996. *Testing the Medical Covenant.* Grand Rapids, MI: Wm. B. Eerdmans Publishing Co., p. 56.

11. Buerki, R.A. 1997. History and human values in ethics instruction. In Haddad, A.M. (Ed.), *Teaching and Learning Strategies in Pharmacy Ethics* (2nd ed.). Binghamton, NY: Pharmaceutical Products Press, imprint of The Haworth Press, Inc., pp. 65–75.

12. Smith, J.F. 1996. Communicative ethics in medicine: The physician patient relationship. In Wolf, S.M. (Ed.), *Feminism and Bioethics.* New York: Oxford University Press, pp. 184–215.

13. Jonsen, A.T. 1990. The good Samaritan as gatekeeper. In *The New Medicine and the Old Ethics.* Cambridge, MA: Harvard University Press, pp. 38–60.

14. Warren, V.L. 1989. Feminist directions in medical ethics. *Hypatia* 4(2):73–87.

15. Moody-Adams, M. 1991. Gender and the complexity of moral voices. In Cord, C. (Ed.), *Feminist Ethics.* Lawrence, KS: University Press of Kansas, pp. 195–212.

16. Sherwin, S. 1992. *No Longer Patient. Feminist Ethics and Health Care.* Philadelphia: Temple University Press.

17. Tong, R. 1993. *Feminine and Feminist Ethics.* Belmont, CA: Wadsworth Publishers.

18. Wolf, S. (Ed.). 1996. *Feminist Bioethics: Beyond Reproduction.* New York: Oxford University Press.

19. Gillett, G. 1997. Is there anything wrong with Hitler these days? Ethics in a post-modern world. *Medical Humanities Review* 11(2):9–20.

20. Dougherty, C., Purtilo, R. 1995. The duty of compassion in an era of healthcare reform. *Cambridge Quarterly* 4:426–433.

21. Peabody, F. 1987 [1927]. The care of the patient. In Stoeckle, J. (Ed.), *Encounters between Patients and Doctors: An Anthology.* Cambridge, MA: MIT Press, pp. 387–401.

22. Barger-Lux, M.J., Heaney, R.P. 1986. For better or worse: The technological imperative in health care. *Social Sciences and Medicine* 22:1313–1320.

23. Poplin, C., Ferrara, J., Cassel, E., et al. 1996. Healing American health care. *The Wilson Quarterly* 20:2.

24. Purtilo, R. 1994. Interdisciplinary health care teams and health care reform. *Journal of Law Medicine and Ethics* 22(2):121–128.

25. Gadow, S. 1985. Nurse and patient: The caring relationship. In Bishop, A.M., Sudder, J.R., Jr. (Eds.), *Caring, Curing, Coping: Nurse, Physician, Patient Relationships.* Birmingham: University of Alabama, pp. 31–43.

26. Jameton, A. 1984. *Nursing Practice: Ethical Issues.* Englewood Cliffs, NJ: Prentice Hall.

27. Fry, S., Killen, A.R., Robinson, E.M. 1996. Care-based reasoning, caring and the ethic of care: A need for clarity. *Journal of Clinical Ethics* 7(1):41–47.

28. Benner, P., Wrubel, J. 1989. *The Primacy of Caring.* Menlo Park, CA: Addison-Wesley.

29. Ruddick, S. 1989. *Maternal Thinking: Toward a Politics of Peace*. Boston: Beacon Press.
30. Condon, E.H. 1991. Nursing and the caring metaphor: Gender and political influences on an ethics of care. *Nursing Outlook* 40(1):14–19.
31. Jonsen, A.L., Toulmin, S. 1988. *The Abuse of Casuistry: A History of Moral Reasoning*. Berkeley: University of California Press.

3

All You Need to Know about Ethics Approaches and Theories—II: Means, Ends, Principles, and Virtues

Objectives

The student should be able to:

- Describe the basic difference between deontological and utilitarian ethical theories.
- Define "right" as it is understood in ethics and law.
- Distinguish freedom rights from entitlement rights.
- Describe the function of a principle (norm, element).
- Identify six principles encountered in professional ethics.
- Compare two ways of interpreting the principles of nonmaleficence and beneficence and discuss how they are used in health care.
- Discuss the meaning of autonomy in Kant's and Mill's theories and the relevance of each to ethical conduct.
- List five reasonable expectations a patient or client has because of the health professional's responsibility to act with fidelity.
- Describe the principle of veracity as it applies in the professional context.
- Compare three aspects of the principle of justice: distributive, compensatory, and procedural.
- Distinguish among absolute, prima facie, and conditional duties or rights.
- Describe the role of moral character or virtue in the realization of a good life.
- List at least six important virtues in Western societies.
- Describe at least six character traits or virtues that are emphasized in ethics codes of the health professions.

New Terms and Ideas You Will Encounter in This Chapter

Deontology	Fidelity
Reason	Veracity
Intuition	Justice—distributive, compensatory,
Teleology	procedural
Utilitarianism	Absolute duties and rights
Principles or elements	Prima facie duties and rights
Nonmaleficence	Conditional duties and rights
Beneficence	Character trait
Autonomy	Virtue and virtues
Rule utilitarian	Moral character

Topics in This Chapter Introduced in Earlier Chapters

TOPIC	INTRODUCED IN	DISCUSSED IN THIS CHAPTER ON
Hippocratic Oath	Chapter 1	Pages 51, 62
The story of Mr. and Mrs. Harvey	Chapter 1	Pages 47, 52, 61
The story of Ronald Rachels	Chapter 2	Pages 47, 53, 58–59
Deductive reasoning	Chapter 2	Page 47

Introduction

In Chapter 1 you were introduced to some basic reasons why ethical reflection is a crucial component of your professional life. In Chapter 2 you began your serious study of approaches designed to help you analyze ethical problems, resolve conflicts, and move to action. In the approaches so far the story (or case) has been the starting point of ethical reflection. In these approaches it has been the end point, too, because with the exception of casuistry (which looks for common themes among cases) you cannot expect any additional resource to help you complete your moral judgment.

The ethical theories you will be working with in this chapter are the more traditional approaches developed in the disciplines of *philosophy* and the parts of *theology* that deal with human values and duties (i.e., issues of morality). If you wish to review the basic definition of morality before proceeding, return to page 7. Three major theories emerge: deontological, utilitarian, and virtue theories. These theories were the bread and butter of professional ethics for many years; therefore you should learn them well. You also will be introduced to several guiding elements or principles. All are helpful, and they also are used most often in ethics writings, discussion, and as the basis for practices, policies, and laws.

THE STORY OF MS DIGRAZIA, MR. HIU, AND THE NEEDLESTICK INCIDENT

Although Ms Angela DiGrazia, a phlebotomist, has worked in the hemophilia clinic for seven years, she has known Mr. Hiu for only a year. Mr. Hiu moved to town a year ago to take a position in a local company. Diagnosed at birth with classic hemophilia A–factor 8 deficiency, he has been a frequenter of hemophilia clinics during his 28 years of life and was relieved to encounter a phlebotomist as good as Angela DiGrazia. Mr. Hiu judges that he has had blood drawn hundreds of times.

Mr. Hiu suffers from acute anxiety attacks when he thinks about the possibility of having received the AIDS virus in a transfusion during the time before safety precautions were tightened.

For the past month Mr. Hiu had been fighting a winter cold. Then ten days ago he became much worse and was hospitalized with symptoms of pneumonia.

Angela has enjoyed talking with Mr. Hiu during his clinic visits. She is visiting a relative who has been admitted to the hospital when she remembers learning he is quite ill and also is a patient here. She decides to drop by to say hello.

During her visit a phlebotomist friend comes in to take a blood sample. She watches while her friend struggles to get into Mr. Hiu's scarred vein. Eager to help, Angela instinctively reaches down to apply pressure to the area and the needle slips. She springs back in alarm and sees blood forming on the spot where the needle has pierced the tip of her forefinger.

Angela immediately asks Mr. Hiu if he would be willing to get tested for HIV to ascertain the risk this injury might incur for her. She knows that in this state the patient is not legally bound to submit automatically to such testing even though the hospital admissions consent form gives patients an opportunity to give such consent at the time they are admitted. (Patients actually are *encouraged* to sign the consent form.) Mr. Hiu abstains, however, saying it is unnecessary because he was found free of the HIV virus two years ago during voluntary testing.

Later that afternoon Angela goes back to Mr. Hiu's room and tells him she thinks it is his moral duty to relieve her of the suffering this accident has caused her. She appeals to him on the basis of a duty to submit to another AIDS test and allow her to know the results.

Is she right? _____ Why or why not? _____

The following additional interesting questions may guide your thinking about the ethical issues in this situation:

Do patients have duties toward health professionals?

If there is a mandate for *patients* to be tested in high-risk situations and the results made known to the professionals treating such patients, should there also be a mandate for *professionals* to be tested and the results made known to their patients? Why does this justice argument make sense—or not make sense—to you?

In this case, if Angela is unsuccessful in persuading Mr. Hiu to consent to testing, would it be morally permissible for her to secretly arrange with the pathology laboratory to do an HIV test on Mr. Hiu's blood as long as all of the other tests that were ordered are done also? If so, who should pay for the testing regimen?

Many would say that Angela should have known better than to endanger her own health by trying to help her friend. Does this change the moral situation she now finds herself in? Why or why not?

There are many theories that address the questions posed in the preceding paragraph. Two conduct-related normative theories that have great relevance for the analysis of moral issues and problems in health care are deontological and teleological theories.

Let us briefly review the meanings of deonto and telos. The root word "deonto" means duty in Greek. The root word "telos" means end.

Which theory would hold, "The ends justify the means"? _____ If you answered, "teleological," you are getting the idea fast. If you have no recollection of these distinctions, return to Chapter 2, page 29, for a quick review.

Following the same line of reasoning, you could say that in deontological theories the _____ justify the _____.

In your daily life you probably rely on a number of expressions to convey your experiences related to conduct you feel some obligation to undertake:

- I ought to.
- I should.
- I have to.
- I must.

When your conduct is geared to ways you think you can help people live together peacefully and harmoniously, the ought or should expressions are attempts to describe deep-seated beliefs about morality and what it requires.

Both deontologists and teleologists express the need for individuals' or groups' actions to be guided accordingly. The deontologist would say that the correct way for you to proceed is to familiarize yourself with the basic duties and rights of individuals or groups and to act in accordance with those guidelines. The teleologist would counter that in some instances adherence to duties or rights might lead to consequences that are contrary to the well-being of a society or the individuals in it. Therefore only when the potential consequences are taken into account can you determine the right course of action.

DEONTOLOGICAL THEORIES

In Chapter 1 Mr. Harvey's health professionals are in a difficult position regarding Mr. Harvey's further treatment for his stroke. In Chapter 2 Ron

Rachels faces a perplexing dilemma regarding loyalty and honesty. In this chapter, Angela DiGrazia is appealing to the patient to respond to her fear. An important task they all share is identifying whether there is a duty that will help them analyze which type of action is morally justifiable under these difficult circumstances.

One place where such factors are presented or codified are in statements that comprise codes of professional ethics. For example, today you will find such statements as, "respect a patient's dignity" or "honor the patient's [or client's] right to consent to a potential treatment." When you look more closely, the statements or axioms imply fundamental ideas about humans, namely that we stand in relation to each other in a number of morally significant ways. In this regard, deontologists agree with Gilligan and others you met in Chapter 2 regarding the centrality of *relationship* and the importance of paying attention to the details of a patient's (or another's) story. But this is as far as their agreement goes. Deontology, unlike the approaches in Chapter 2, holds that there are basic concepts individuals and societies recognize and agree upon that give rise to a shared sense of duty or right. These could be arrived at through *reasoning* about such things, or others might argue, we *intuit* them (i.e., have intuition; note the deductive assumptions discussed in the beginning of Chapter 2). Although a narrative approach correctly helps to focus attention on particular details of a story, the deontologist goes further to say there is in fact a concept of duty informing (or at least available to) all individuals.

Deontological theories hold that you are acting rightly when you act according to duties and rights. Responsibility arises from these moral facts of life. In other words, duties and rights are the correct measuring rods for evaluating action. There are many versions of these deductive reasoning theories. The person most often identified with deontological approaches is Immanuel Kant (1724–1804). His basic premises still figure strongly in arguments within health care ethics today. He held that every person has an inherent dignity and on that basis alone is entitled to respect. Respect is shown by never *using* people to achieve goals or consequences. He thought that duties and rights help to determine how respect toward others can be expressed. It follows that the morally correct thing is always to be guided by moral duties, rights, and responsibilities. He concluded that some actions are intrinsically immoral, no matter how positive and beneficial one might judge the consequences to be, and that other actions are intrinsically moral, no matter how negative the consequences might be. In short, he said that one cannot judge the moral rightness or wrongness of an act on the basis of its consequences alone.[1] Although his conclusion about whether Mr. Hiu should submit to the HIV test is not self-evident, Kant would arrive at his decision by a process of determining what his duty should be, not simply whether there would be overall better consequences by one type of act or another.

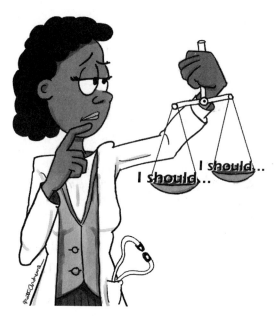

FIGURE 3–1 Weighing duties.

As you can begin to see, some challenges are inherent in this approach. For instance, the idea that we ought to do the right thing, informed by duty, is general. *How* to show respect for individuals still needs further interpretation in any situation. What do we do when duties or rights themselves come into conflict? Deontological theories require that a method of weighing be available to determine what to do when conflicts arise, and critics charge that there is no obvious way to weigh them. Such a process is not self-evident. As you will see in a later discussion in this chapter, the appeal to *principles* is one attempt to provide further detail and interpretation to the general idea of duty and to order, or give varying weight to, various duties, rights, and responsibilities.

TELEOLOGICAL THEORIES

Partially because of some of the criticisms of deontology, *teleological theories* emerged, placing the focus on consequences of actions. The most important teleological theory for our consideration of health care ethics is *utilitarianism*. This word takes its root from the idea of *utility* or usefulness.

In utilitarianism an act is right if it helps to bring about the best balance of benefits over burdens, in other words, the best consequences overall. This approach was developed first by two English philosophers, Jeremy Bentham (1748–1832)[2] and John Stuart Mill (1860–1873).[3] You will note that they are roughly contemporaries of Kant. In fact, they were vigorous opponents of Kant's position.

Consider Angela DiGrazia's request. How will you decide what Mr. Hiu should do? What she should do? From a utilitarian point of view, first you must consider what several different courses of action could accomplish. You might say something like, "The goal is to treat Mr. Hiu in such a way that everyone else will be able to have the same type of treatment he is receiving," or, "The goal is to be able to live with my own conscience." If both these goals can be attained by taking one, single course of action, it should be taken. If this is not possible, the course of action you believe will bring about the best consequences overall should take priority.

One important task of this approach is to distinguish alternative paths of action and then predict as accurately as possible the consequences of each path. As you can begin to see, this approach, too, has some inherent challenges. How can anyone predict all the potential consequences of an act? Moreover, doesn't this approach ignore the fact that at least sometimes humans do think in terms of their duties, rights, and responsibilities to one another?

DUTIES AND CONSEQUENCES IN TENSION

The deontological and utilitarian normative theories have been helpful to health professionals because they set a general framework for thinking about specific moral issues and problems in health care settings. Probably as you were reading you were thinking, "Well, both the idea of duties and rights *and* the idea of consequences are important." In fact, most of us do draw on both to make practical, everyday decisions. Only occasionally does it make a big difference in what you judge to be right if you follow a deontological line of reasoning or appeal to consequences only. Fortunately, most of the time you can follow your duty, honor others' rights, *and* consider the consequences you are bringing about without any conflict among the three. But it is in the occasional moment at which the means and the ends seem to be competing that it will become necessary to plant your feet firmly in one approach or the other and be able to justify why.

For your review, here are the two theories:

DEONTOLOGY	TELEOLOGY
duty-driven	goal-driven
means count	ends count
Kant	Bentham, Mill (utilitarians)

As you work your way through this book, continue to reflect on your position regarding these two major theories and why you think it best serves you in your goal to live a moral life.

PRINCIPLES AS GUIDES: HOW TO EXPRESS RESPECT FOR OTHERS

As the preceding discussions suggest, a serious shortcoming of using deontological or utilitarian theory as the sole tool for everyday ethical decision making is the generality of each: each provides a broad canvas upon which further details for action could be painted. Many ethicists have pondered over this concern, and from further development of the basic theories, certain useful norms or *elements* to guide action that expresses respect for the dignity of human beings have been identified. In most professional ethics literature as well as modern social ethics writings they are called *principles*. I also think of them as *elements* because they do for ethical theory what the basic chemical elements do for chemistry theory: they provide a way to see something concretely that is quite abstract. As you know, a chemical element can be combined with other elements. Sometimes they combine to form a new compound that looks and acts differently than each of the units taken individually. Sometimes they clash. Often two or more elements have different relative weights so that one is heavier than the other(s). You will be introduced to each in some detail. They are shown in Table 3–1 for your future reference.

TABLE 3–1 Ethical Principles

Principle	When Applicable
Nonmaleficence (refraining from potentially harming myself or another)	I am in a position to harm someone else.
Beneficence (bringing about good)	I am in a position to benefit someone else.
Fidelity	I have made a promise, explicit or implicit, to someone else.
Autonomy	I have an opportunity to exercise my freedom in a situation.
Veracity	I am in a position to tell the truth or deceive someone.
Justice	I am in a position to distribute benefits and burdens among individuals or groups in society who have legitimate claims on the benefits.

There is more to the story than Table 3–1 indicates because "I" may be a person, a group, or even an institution. Principles can help you know how an individual, group, or institution stands in relationship to other people, morally speaking. The British philosopher David Hume justified this position in his belief that we incur obligations to act in certain ways because we have received positive responses to our own needs and expectations of being treated humanely: "I have benefitted from society, and therefore ought to promote its interests."[4] Some philosophers argue, correctly I think, that principles help to identify what we should do in special relationships regardless of whether we have received benefits from the other person (or from society). Some such relationships are between parent and child, health professional and patient, spouses, faculty and student, lawyer and client, or citizen and society.

As you continue to read you will discover more fully why deontologists and utilitarians may both find the idea of principles helpful but that principles play a somewhat different role in each theory: The deontologist, guided by duty, views principles as more specific delineations of duties (or rights). A utilitarian weighs the consequences of acting according to the various principles and discerns which one (or ones) will bring about the most favorable (or least damaging) consequences overall in a situation.

In Chapter 4 we will go into more detail about how principles sometimes come into conflict in a situation. It is not a perfect world, and ethical conflicts do arise. Although the final decision about what to do might be the same for a deontologist and utilitarian, the deontologist would bear more burden of guilt about the decision if acting on one principle meant compromising another. For him or her, compromising any principle is wrong, although at times it is necessary to choose the lesser of two evils. The utilitarian would resolve the conflict by choosing the best consequences that could be brought about, although he, too, may realize it is not a perfect situation.

Several principles are extremely important in the health care context. For example, the principle of nonmaleficence or, in everyday language, "do no harm," was an explicit theme in the ancient Hippocratic Oath and ever since has been viewed as an overriding moral principle guiding health professionals' conduct toward patients. Because of their importance you have this opportunity to examine several in more detail.

Nonmaleficence and Beneficence

Primum non nocere (First, do no harm) is thought to be at the nexus of traditional health care ethics and often is attributed to the author of the Hippocratic Oath. The principle of *nonmaleficence* is the noun used today to talk about this type of action. You can figure out the general meaning of the term by breaking it into its prefix, non, and the root, maleficence (mal, bad or evil). The difference in power between professional and patient alone helps to support the instinctive wisdom of this strong call to refrain from abuse. Furthermore, Western societies in general usually attribute greater significance to a harmful act that requires deliberate intent than to one done out of neglect or ignorance. It is difficult to believe that a society could survive if people went around trying to harm each other, and the laws of our land take seriously the necessity of stemming the potential for harm to go unchecked. The early purveyors of professional ethics left nothing to chance, warning health professionals that there was no room whatsoever for acting in ways designed to bring about harm.

In professional ethics, not harming and acting to benefit another are treated as separate duties, with not harming as the more compelling moral element driving decision making. Sometimes, however, philosophers treat them as different levels of the same principle or element. When duties are thought of in this fashion, at least four types fall along the continuum of the same principle:

Do no harm.
Prevent harm.
Remove harm when it is being inflicted.
Bring about positive good.

Professional ethics limits *beneficence* to the last three on the list but agrees that this type of behavior, too, is extremely important. Put succinctly, Beauchamp and Childress claim that "X has a positive duty of beneficence towards Y when X has the capacity to promote Y's well-being."[5]

This is an apt moment to think about how deontologists and utilitarians would view beneficence because health professionals will include both types of thinkers: Deontologists hold that beneficence is a _____ (fill in the blank) to bring about positive good in your interaction with patients, clients, and others. At the very least you must strive to act beneficently by preventing and removing harm when the opportunity arises for you to apply your skills, knowledge, and compassion to accomplish this goal. A utilitarian would focus on the _____ (again, fill in the blank). In other words, he would strive to *optimize the amount of positive good*. This goal allows you to understand why observers suggest that the overriding (some theorists say the only) principle that counts in utilitarianism is beneficence. In utilitarianism you must strive to bring about the most good or "benefit" possible in the situation.

To illustrate further, in the story of Mr. Harvey and the health professionals told in Chapter 1, the deontologist would think about "do no harm" and "do what is good for the patient" in terms of specific duties the health professionals have. In terms of their professional role, which specific harms can health professionals refrain from inflicting? Are they in a position to prevent or remove harm? If so, they have a duty to act in those ways. The utilitarian would weigh the possibilities for doing good in the scales to decide which action would bring about the most good overall.

Before you leave the principles of nonmaleficence and beneficence, think again about the story described in Chapter 2. Ron is worried about what has happened to the patient, Pamela Faden. He believes she has been harmed by having a scalpel left in her abdominal cavity and, then, by the surgeon's failure to tell her about the surgical error.

Is Ron following the principle of nonmaleficence by his actions so far? The principle of beneficence? What evidence do you have that he is or is not? In your opinion what would he have to do to be beneficent in this case, given the level of his authority and his knowledge, skills, and compassion?

Finally, consider the story of Ms DiGrazia and Mr. Hiu introduced at the beginning of this chapter. This story raises interesting questions about the relevance of the principles of nonmaleficence and beneficence in different situations. First, Ms DiGrazia was not acting in her professional role when the accident occurred. Health professions' codes of ethics generally are deontological in their approach, but they do not address the duties that patients or society have toward health professionals or other citizens. So there will be little help to guide either Ms DiGrazia or Mr. Hiu within the health professions context per se. She is appealing to Mr. Hiu to submit to a medical test to remove harm (i.e., her anxiety and possible infection) and bring about some good. In society there is a duty (expressed in laws) not to intentionally harm another, but Mr. Hiu did not intentionally harm her, unless you have concluded that his refusal to submit to the test is now causing her harm. Therefore she is appealing to a duty of beneficence, which the law does not recognize except in special situations, and this is *not* one of them.

Because these two principles are so pervasive in the everyday decision making by a professional, you are well advised to think about their relevance in every new situation you encounter.

Autonomy

The principle of *autonomy* is the capacity to have the say-so about your own well-being, "the capacity to think, decide and act on the basis of such thought and decision freely and independently."[6] Some call this the principle of self-determination. Obviously the principle applies to you whether you are acting in your professional role (professional autonomy) or as a citizen (social autonomy) or have become a patient (patient autonomy). Much of the discussion that follows focuses on the important arena of patient autonomy.

We know that patients' basic health care needs have not changed a lot over the decades, but our responses have changed. Today so many clinical interventions are possible that the type and number of interventions alone may lead to suffering. A few years ago the health professional who did every-

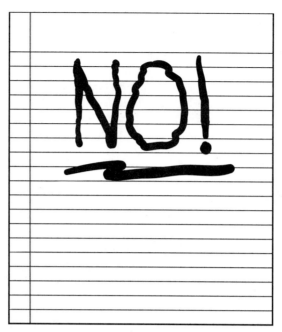

FIGURE 3–2 This statement was written on a pad of paper by a 27-year-old hospitalized woman with ovarian-breast cancer syndrome. She could not communicate verbally because she had a tracheostomy and therefore could not speak. The physician had explained that he wanted to reimplement chemotherapy for a tumor that had appeared in her remaining ovary. She had already undergone an oophorectomy and hysterectomy and had received radiotherapy and chemotherapy for the previous tumors before their removal.

thing clinically possible for a patient was seen as being beneficent. Today that same professional could find that the process leads to regret: The patient or patient's family may charge that harm has resulted because the interventions have been beyond what the patient wanted or could tolerate.

In the light of this situation the past several decades have seen the emergence of the patient as a more active negotiator regarding health care decisions. The patient's *autonomy*, say-so or self-governance, has come to be accepted as a legitimate moral claim to be placed in the balance with the health professional's independent judgment about what is beneficent.

The principle of autonomy (or self-determination) and its role in morality have been developed from the views of such diverse and colorful figures in philosophy as Kant, Sarte, Mill, and Hare. The preeminent deontologist, Immanuel Kant, whom you have met before, and one of the crafters of utilitarianism, John Stuart Mill, were particularly instrumental in shaping the concept of autonomy, and both of their interpretations have been adopted in the principle of autonomy as it is used in the health professions today. Kant emphasized the role of being in control of making one's own choices in accord with principles that could be willed to be valid for everyone.[7] Therefore, his main contribution to the principle of autonomy was his discussion of self-legislation: the reasons for actions. Conversely, Mill focused his thought more on the context of the freedom of action, arguing that an individual's actions legitimately are constricted only when they promise to harm someone else. Up to that point, he contends, each person should be permitted to act according to his or her own convictions. Therefore his main contribution was to highlight the social and political context in which the exercise of autonomy can be realized.[8]

The two interpretations together point to our belief that a patient's input can be rational and that the context of decision making must be conducive to the patient's exercising his or her real and informed wishes.

Gilligan (see Chapter 2), among others, criticizes a focus on autonomy because it requires that a person be treated as an isolated unit standing alone, over and against all other people, whereas she emphasizes the importance of relationship for the moral life.[9] This is a serious criticism. She is correct in her observation that we understand ourselves as moral beings largely within the context of our relationships. Be that as it may, we do live in a society that is highly individualistic in its behavior and laws.[10] The principle of autonomy provides direction in those situations in which an individual is in a position to make a claim on others to respect his or her selfhood. In fact, sometimes the claim for autonomy is given the power of a right.

Today there is a lot of discussion about autonomy in regard to decisions about the timing and type of death one will have. Underlying the idea of a right to die is the more fundamental belief in the right to autonomy or self-determination. This, too, has arisen at least partly out of the predicament society is in as a result of the myriad clinical interventions available. Sometimes a patient has just had enough, but the health professional feels bound to keep providing treatments, believing it to be beneficent to do so, because they are available.

The principle of autonomy has much broader applications than end-of-life situations. In the predicament Mr. Hiu finds himself in at the beginning of this chapter there is not full consensus about whose wishes should prevail in regard to his being tested for his present HIV status. What do you think?

His autonomy should govern because _____

_____ ;

  or

Ms DiGrazia's autonomy should govern because _____

_____ .

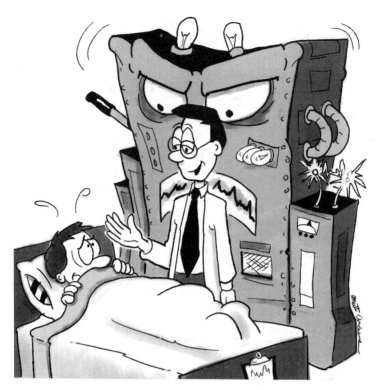

FIGURE 3–3

Do you think John Stuart Mill would agree? Yes _____ No _____
Mill would base his judgment about the limits of Mr. Hiu's autonomy on whether *overall* his being allowed to refrain would be the best consequence that could be brought about in this situation. (A *rule utilitarian** would say that to follow the rule and be kind—beneficent—to a person who is in as much distress as Angela DiGrazia always would bring about better consequences than standing firm on the basis of one's own prerogative or right not to submit to the test.

The principle of self-determination is a helpful principle, but, like all of the principles, it is not absolute in the delicate complexity of real life situations. For example, Mill would put his foot down at the point when one person's exercise of autonomy would lead to the direct harm of another. If I

*Rule utilitarians are sometimes thought of as a hybrid between duty-oriented approaches, which rely on certain forms of actions, and pure utilitarians, who think about consequences solely in the specific details of each situation. A rule utilitarian would hold that you will always bring about more good consequences by following certain rules. What the rules should be then becomes the task for these theorists.

want to hit you, my autonomy ends where your nose begins. Should Mr. Hiu's autonomy end where Angela DiGrazia's pleading begins? This is such a serious issue that laws of different states have ruled differently regarding the extent of Mr. Hiu's autonomy in this type of situation. As with many ethical issues, the relative newness of AIDS and the fear of infection has led to widespread public debate about the right thing to do to respect the ideals of our life together. Within the health professional ethics community there is understandable caution about moving too hastily in the direction of compromising patient self-determination, even in such moments.

You will revisit the principle of autonomy in the discussion of informed consent in Chapter 11, as well as encountering it in the analysis of several ethical issues throughout the rest of this book.

Fidelity

The principle of *fidelity* comes from the Latin root *fides*, which means faithfulness. Being faithful to the patient entails meeting the patient's reasonable expectations. The patients come with all kinds of expectations. What can be counted as a *reasonable* expectation?

First, there are reasonable expectations that basic respect will be shown to anyone, anywhere. Sometimes health professionals have been criticized for failing to show basic respect, like respecting the modesty of a patient.

Second, the patient has reason to expect that you will be competent in what you do.

Third, the patient has a reasonable expectation that you will adhere to statements you have subscribed to as a member of a profession. The most public of these statements is your code of ethics. Take it out again and see what your professional code says.

Fourth, the patient has a good basis for believing you will follow the policies and statements adopted by your place of employment, as well as laws that are designed to protect patients' well-being.

Finally, the patient has good reason to expect that you will honor what the two of you have agreed to, such as the promises involved in any informed consent form the patient has signed, verbal agreements, or serious conversations.

Can you think of others?

Veracity

The ethical element of *veracity* binds you to honesty. Veracity means that you will tell the truth. This principle is more specific than, say, beneficence or fidelity. For this reason some would call it a second level principle directing you to engage in a specific type of behavior, which in turn can support your intent to be beneficent or to maintain your fidelity in relationship to patients and others. Immanuel Kant, the philosopher you met earlier in this chapter, gave veracity a more central role than most thinkers, taking the position that veracity is an absolute to which no exception can be made "however great may be the disadvantage accruing to yourself or another." The lie, he argues in one place, always is wrong because the practice of lying is something that weakens the entire human fabric.[1] Most others would weigh veracity heavily regarding its potential for benefiting others but would not make it the absolute or governing duty above all others.

In the story presented in Chapter 2, Ron understandably seemed depressed about the possibility that Pamela Faden was not being told the truth about the surgeon's mistake. The situation was made more complex by the different professional roles of the radiologic technologist and the physician. Given his role, do you think that as a radiologic technologist Ron personally should have acted according to the principle of veracity and told her about the scalpel? Do you think that the surgeon had a moral obligation to tell her the truth?

The story of Angela DiGrazia and Mr. Hiu certainly can be analyzed according to this principle. The truth about Mr. Hiu's HIV status lies between them like a wall separating their relationship. If I were to say that for the good of Angela as well as of all humankind Mr. Hiu must take the necessary steps so that she can learn the truth, would you agree? Yes _____ No _____ If not, what other principles would you weigh against veracity in this situation that leads you to your conclusion?

_____

_____

Later in this book we return to the important matter of truth telling as it relates to your professional task of disclosing different types of information in general. In preparation, take a minute to jot down one or two challenging situations in which you can imagine that the truth would be difficult:

_____

_____

_____

Justice

Patients do not always get all the treatment and attention they deserve or need because of a lack of resources, and anyone who worries about that is worrying about the *justice* of the situation. Discrimination against some individuals or groups may appear to be shortchanging them, and anyone who worries about that is worrying about the justice of the situation. A lack of due process regarding who receives priority in situations of conflict may cause concern, and anyone who worries about that also is worrying about the justice of the situation. In general, their concern is that all similarly situated persons receive their fair share of benefits and assume their fair share of burdens.

Justice can be thought of as an arbiter. It is called on when there are problems regarding what is rightfully due a person, institution, or society. Three types of justice have particular importance in professional ethics situations: distributive, compensatory, and procedural.

Distributive Justice

Questions of distributive justice arise when more than one group is competing for the same resources, each believing itself to be deserving of the resources. The principle of distributive justice requires an equitable distribution of benefits and burdens. "Equitable" means that the amount will vary according to different levels of need, or merit, given the situation.

Consider just a few of the many possible ways of spending tax money on health-related procedures. How much should be spent on antismoking campaigns? AIDS research? Improving living conditions in the ghetto? Extensively treating Alzheimer's disease in elderly people? Eradicating birth defects through genetic engineering? Finding a cure for cancer? Developing an artificial heart and making it available to everyone with severe heart disease? Educating health professionals? Developing a better treatment for crack addiction? Finding a vaccine for the common cold? Screening for head lice among school children? Providing funds to make hospitals more humane, caring environments? Conducting research to eradicate malaria? Providing plastic surgery for people who want it?

A search for the best criteria on which to base allocation decisions is the challenge of distributive justice.

Compensatory Justice

Compensatory justice concerns compensations for wrongs that have been done. The compensation does not have to be for a legal or moral wrong suffered by a person. For example, in the case of accidents, there may be an appeal to a notion of compensation: The victim expects aid even though no one can be found guilty of imposing the injury.

Do you think Angela DiGrazia deserves to be compensated for the harm she is experiencing from the needlestick even though Mr. Hiu did not intend to harm her? Yes _____ No _____ If so, what kind of compensation do you suggest, and why?

_____

_____

Compare this situation with that in Chapter 2. Do you think the patient Pamela Faden deserves to be compensated for the harm she has experienced from Dr. Kristansen's mistake, even though he did not intend to harm her? Yes _____ No _____ If so, what kind of compensation do you suggest, and why?

_____

_____

What, if any, is the difference between Angela DiGrazia's claim for compensation and Pamela Faden's, if any?

_____

_____

The question of compensation is raised also regarding groups in society who have been "wronged" because of past discriminations on the basis of race, color, sex, age, or other characteristics. Should they be compensated by receiving priority in medical care allocations?

(Compensatory justice also can be applied to the area of justice dealing with punishment, especially within the context of criminal justice. In this application of the concept, compensation is for a legal or moral wrong and is referred to as "retributive justice.")

Procedural Justice

Questions of procedural justice arise in processes that require ordering in a fair manner. In Western society a "first come, first served" basis is considered fair treatment in many situations. For example, is it fair to treat a patient who arrives at 9:00 for his 9:45 appointment if it is 9:01 and the 9:00 patient has not arrived?

Impartiality is a key concept in pure procedural justice. Policies often are designed to assure that the same procedures apply to all comers. As a thought experiment try to develop a policy to cover the situation described in the preceding paragraph and also to identify which types of justice (and other principles) you had to include in order to decide how this situation should be handled.

Absolute, Prima Facie, and Conditional Principles

Before leaving this lengthy discussion of principles, consider three basic distinctions regarding them: Principles that carry the weight of duties or rights may be absolute, prima facie, or conditional. *Absolute* duties or rights are binding under all circumstances. They can never give way to another compelling duty or right. *Prima facie* duties or rights allow you to make choices among conflicting principles. For instance, the prima facie duty of veracity is actually binding if it conflicts with no other duties, or rights, that are weightier in a given situation. But it is not an element that is absolute either, since other elements may be more compelling. In the discussion of the primacy of "do no harm" over "beneficience" in the clinical ethics context, it was suggested that each is being treated as a prima facie principle, and the mandate not to harm is more compelling than the mandate to bring about some positive good. A *conditional duty* is a commitment that comes into being only after certain conditions are met. For example, the United States' Americans with Disabilities Act[11] outlines certain legal rights and responsibilities that apply solely to persons who have disabilities. The goal was to base the document on moral duties and rights.

However binding a principle or element is deemed to be, it shares the role of providing a marker for conduct to persons and groups wanting to live a good moral life. Three prototypes of ethical problems in which principles may conflict, and a method for dealing with each, are discussed in Chapter 4. But before you continue on to ethical problem solving, there is one more important type of ethical theory to address.

VIRTUE THEORY

We have surmised that Mr. Hiu's intent is not to cause Angela harm: he simply does not want to consider whether he has a duty to be HIV tested for her benefit or whether he should go the additional mile, beyond his duty, to help her. What kind of a person would make these choices? In this final section of the chapter you will be introduced to character traits and the role of the virtues in actions.

Character Traits and Moral Character

A *character trait* is a disposition or a readiness to act in certain ways. Some people exhibit character traits that lead an observer to judge that they are of a *high moral character*. In other words, they are a type of person who can be *expected* always to act in a manner that will be praised by others because it upholds high standards. To some extent, our society is measured by the type of people in it.

Certain character traits enable you to be the kind of person you want to be as a caregiver.[12] For example, honesty will manifest itself in your trying to refrain from deceiving others for your own comfort or protection. Courage may be required to speak out against injustice or other wrongdoing. Courage combined with honesty will be needed for a nurse to admit that she or he mistakenly gave the wrong medication to a patient. Compassion can help motivate you to refrain from thoughtlessly harming vulnerable people.

Remember the health professionals involved in Mr. Harvey's care? Honesty taken alone might dispose you to fill out Mr. Harvey's medical forms in a way that would not deceive anyone (but unfortunately would also lead to his premature discharge from your unit). Honesty and courage taken together may dispose you to fill out the form as above but try to help change a system that has placed both of you in an unfair bind. These two character traits combined with compassion might motivate you to express your sympathy to the Harvey family as well. In each case a character trait has enabled activity that can be respected, even when the outcome is not ideal. Taken together, the habitual practice of exercising these traits creates a high moral character that prompts you to do everything possible to diminish the amount of harm.

Over the centuries the importance attached to various character traits has varied. For instance, the ancient Greek traits of wisdom, temperance, courage, and justice still are widely cherished. In Western society the early Christian church accepted these Greek traits while adding their own Christian virtues of faith, hope, and love. The Puritan motive of industriousness ("busy hands are happy hands") is deeply embedded in our value systems. Honesty, loving kindness, and reasonableness often are named. As you learned in Chapter 2, some writers in the health professions emphasize character traits related to caring. In Chapter 12 you will have an opportunity to examine the critical character trait of compassion.

These attitudes, traits, and motives often are referred to as *virtues* in ethical writings. Failure to exhibit basic moral character or virtue will cause an individual to be judged (morally) blameworthy or unvirtuous.

The importance of moral character has been affirmed in many major health professions writings, historically and today. For example, authors of the Hippocratic school wrote approximately 70 essays on health care in addition to the Oath. Several discussed character traits. The *Decorum* enjoins that a physician should be modest, sober, patient, prompt, and conduct himself with propriety in professional and personal life.[13] In short, the caregiver will have the moral fiber required to carry out the various duties outlined in the Oath.

Maimonides was a highly respected and renowned Jewish philosopher of the thirteenth century who wrote extensively on the relationship of medical issues to Jewish law. The prayer of Maimonides is based directly on the belief that the development of certain character traits or virtues enables the caregiver to exhibit appropriate moral behavior. In making this promise the physician calls on God for help to have the right motives, worthy of this high calling:

> May neither avarice nor miserliness, nor thirst for glory, nor for great reputation, engage my mind, or the enemies of truth and philanthropy could easily deceive me and make me forgetful of my lofty aim of doing good to my patients. May I never see in a patient anything but a fellow creature of pain.[14]

Maimonides believed that important character traits of the health professional are sympathy for the patient's plight, humility, and a devoted commitment to helping others.

Many suggestions regarding the need for high moral character citeu ... the preceding examples are implied in the modern codes of ethics of the health professions. Examine the code of your chosen health field. What character traits are listed or implied? Probably the most widely esteemed traits are those that convey an attitude of respect for persons who come to you as patients. The underlying ideal is that individuals should be treated as ends, not as means to some other end.

An important, and sometimes overlooked, aspect of treating people as ends is related to the difference in power that exists between caregivers and patients. Because the caregiver almost always has more information about the illness, knows more about the treatment, and can make a difference in the life of the patient in concrete ways, to some extent the patient (or the subject of a medical research project) is always at the mercy of the practitioner. Although much can be done to include the patient in decision making, this power differential almost always exists. In the final analysis the quality of care and the extent to which the patient is treated with dignity largely rest on the type of people who deliver health care services.

A similar sentiment was expressed by the patient who said of her long-term hospitalization that she had no complaints whatsoever about the treatment she received and that she was included in her treatment planning, but

> I've seen a lot of . . . action these last two months, and I think I've seen a lot of things. . . .
> Now for instance, many patients have got to be moved. They're constantly moving them because of bed sores and different things. Well, some of them will come along and you'd really think they were dealing with a leg of lamb or cattle or something. I think there is such a thing as being a bit humane with a patient.[15]

In recent years ethicists have begun to speak of the virtues of institutions, an issue you will encounter more fully in Chapter 7.

In short, both individual and institutional virtues are important within the health professions. In this respect one can speak of the moral character of an individual health professional as well as the moral character of health care institutions. More will be said about both in later chapters of this book.

SUMMARY

This chapter introduces you to the most important principles or norms of ethics that you need to understand the ethical aspects of your life as a professional person. Duties and rights will help you to have the conceptual tools for recognizing and working to resolve problems that arise in your everyday practice. The development of moral character will help you be ready for the hard times when no answers seem to be forthcoming or when you are confronted with something that is not easy to face. Although traditionally much of the language of health care ethics has been that of what is owed the patient (i.e., the language of duties), more recently the ideas of patients' (as well as professionals' and society's) rights and the importance of character traits and attitudes have enriched the understanding of this aspect of practice. With this basic framework at your disposal you are well positioned to examine the four prototypical ethical problems you will face.

Questions for Thought and Discussion

1. Describe two situations that may arise in your future professional career that illustrate the ethical dimensions of your conduct as a health professional.

2. Cite an example from health care in which a conflict could arise between your sense of duty to the patient and the negative consequences your act might have on someone else.

3. Elva, a 370-pound, 62-year-old woman, is in a nursing home following complications of diabetes and several small strokes. Although she has been obese all her life, she now is at a weight where it is impossible to move her without a lift. Elva, however, refuses to be moved by it, claiming, "I'm not a piece of meat."

   It is possible to transfer her to a chair using four or five of the staff. The administration, however, is worried that the staff could be injured while moving her physically. Her daughter insists that it is a violation of Elva's dignity as well as an unnecessary compromise of her autonomy to submit her to "the indignity of the mechanical lift."

   You are the supervisor of the unit. What ethical guidelines presented in Chapter 3 can help you to assess what to do in this situation? What should you do?

4. Walter is a resident in the same nursing home with Elva. He is a 78-year-old widower who has been on antidepressants since the sudden death of his wife five years ago. He, too, is visited often by his daughter. The staff of the nursing home inadvertently threw out his dentures with the sheets while making his bed. He had a habit of leaving them on the bed, and although the staff usually noticed them, a new person failed to do so.

   Since then, Walter has adamantly refused to have his teeth replaced. The nursing home administration is more than willing to fit him with a new set of dentures and to pay all costs. His daughter is very much in agreement with the administration that he should have his teeth replaced. They are all aware that his nutrition is suffering as well as his ability to be understood when he tries to talk.

Should Walter be allowed to continue without his dentures? What principles and other considerations of ethics should you, as a nursing home administrator, bring to bear on your decision on how to proceed in this situation? What should you do?

References

1. Kant, I. 1949. In Beck, L.W. (Ed.), *Critique of Practical Reason and other Writings in Moral Philosophy*. Chicago: University of Chicago Press, pp. 346–350.
2. Bentham, J. 1939. In Burtt, E.A. (Ed.), *The English Philosophers from Bacon to Mill*. New York: Random House, pp. 792–856.
3. Mill, J.S. 1939. Utilitarianism. In Burtt, E.A. (Ed.), *The English Philosophers from Bacon to Mill*. New York: Random House, pp. 895–1041.
4. Hume, D. 1976. On suicide. In Gorowitz, S., et al. (Eds.). *Moral Problems in Medicine*. Englewood Cliffs, NJ: Prentice Hall, p. 356.
5. Beauchamp, T., Childress, J.F. 1994. *Principles of Biomedical Ethics* (4th ed.). New York: Oxford University Press, pp. 259–260.
6. Gillon, R. 1994. *Philosophical Medical Ethics*. Chichester, England: John Wiley, p. 60.
7. Kant, I. 1963. *Lectures on Ethics* (translated by Louis Infield). New York: Harper and Row, pp. 147–154.
8. Mill, J.S. 1939. On Liberty. In Burtt, E.A. (Ed.), *The English Philosophers from Bacon to Mill*. pp. 1042–1060.
9. Gilligan, C. 1982. *Psychological Theory and Women's Development*. Cambridge, MA: Harvard University Press.
10. Bellah, R., et al. 1985. *Habits of the Heart: Individualism and Commitment in American Life*. Berkeley, CA: University of California Press.
11. Americans with Disabilities Act. 1990. H.R. Rep. No. 485 (II), 101st Congress, 2nd Sess. at 22 12.
12. Loewy, E.H. 1997. Developing habits and knowing what habits to develop: A look at the role of virtue in ethics. *Cambridge Quarterly Healthcare Ethics* 6(3):347–355.
13. Hippocrates. Decorum. In *Hippocrates II* (translation by W.H.S. Jones), Loeb Classical Library. Cambridge, MA: Harvard University Press, pp. 267–302.
14. Maimonides. 1927. Prayers of Moses Maimonides (translated by H. Friedenwald). *Bulletin of the Johns Hopkins Hospital* 28:260–261.
15. Langone, J. 1974. *Vital Signs*. Boston: Little, Brown, p. 309.

4

Prototypes of Ethical Problems

Objectives

The student should be able to:
- Identify and explain three prototypical ethical problems.
- Describe what an "agent" is and, more importantly, what it is to be a *"moral agent."*
- Describe the role of emotions and character traits in ethical distress.
- Compare the fundamental difference between ethical distress and an ethical dilemma.
- Define ethical paternalism or parentalism.
- Describe the key components of an ethical dilemma that challenges justice.
- Identify the fundamental difference between distress or dilemma problems and locus of authority problems.
- Identify four aspects of professional life that may have bearing on the decision about who should assume authority for various decisions.

New Terms and Ideas You Will Encounter in This Chapter

Moral agent	Integrity	Paternalism/parentalism
Ethical distress	Ethical dilemma	Locus of authority problem

Topics in This Chapter Introduced in Earlier Chapters

TOPIC	INTRODUCED IN	DISCUSSED IN THIS CHAPTER ON
Ethical issue	Chapter 1	Page 67
Ethical problem	Chapter 1	Page 67
Applied ethics	Chapter 1	Page 70
Story of Ronald Rachels	Chapter 2	Page 74
Role of emotions	Chapter 2	Page 71
Deontology	Chapter 3	Page 73

Topic	Introduced In	Discussed In This Chapter On
Utilitarianism	Chapter 3	Pages 73, 74
Elements/principles	Chapter 3	Page 73
Beneficence	Chapter 3	Page 73
Autonomy	Chapter 3	Page 74
Fidelity	Chapter 3	Page 73
Character traits	Chapter 3	Pages 71, 72
Principles	Chapter 3	Page 74

Introduction

In *The Magic Mountain*, Thomas Mann notes that "order and simplification are the first steps toward the mastery of a subject."[1] With the fundamentals of ethics with which you will be working having been set out, this chapter introduces you to three prototypes of ethical problems. They are summarized in the box below. Each will help to order and simplify the material you have encountered so far and will give you a much better idea of how to apply the various theories and approaches to your everyday experience. You may recall that two basic notions introduced in Chapter 1 were an ethical issue and an ethical problem.

An *ethical issue* is a situation that you believe may have important moral values and duties embedded in it that you want to identify. They are present but do not necessarily create a problem.

An *ethical problem* is a situation that you have reason to think presents serious challenges or threats to important moral values and duties. The situation requires you to reflect on what type of person you should be or on what you should do.

In this chapter the focus on ethical problems signals that they will give you difficulty in your everyday life as a professional. See the following three prototypes of problems in ethics:

- **Ethical distress:** You face a challenge about how to maintain your integrity or the integrity of the profession.
- **Ethical dilemma:** You face a challenge about the morally right thing to do; two courses of action diverge.
- **Locus of authority problem:** You face the challenge of deciding who should be the primary decision maker.

The following story sets the stage for our discussion:

THE STORY OF TIFFANY BRYANT AND BEULAH WATSON

Beulah Watson is a 46-year-old environmental services employee in a large hotel in town. She has been employed for 18 years in this position and by and large says she has enjoyed her work. In recent years, however, she has increasingly suffered from shoulder and elbow pain that Dr. Chou, the rheumatologist in the hotel's health plan, accredits to her many years of tugging and hauling heavy linens and cleaning equipment required in the course of her work.

Tiffany Bryant is the occupational therapist who has been treating Ms Watson for the pain and stiffness that has caused her so much discomfort and increased her absenteeism. Beulah Watson originally was very prompt in keeping her appointments, but recently she has missed almost all of her sessions. Tiffany is concerned about whether Beulah is taking the time off to do other things while telling her workplace that she has a therapy appointment. This idea starts to work on Tiffany, and she gets more and more annoyed with Beulah.

Finally Tiffany calls the hotel environmental services manager. She tells her about Beulah's missed appointments (five in the last six weeks). She also tells the manager that the hotel's health plan is being charged for the missed visits, that being the policy of the institution where Tiffany is employed.

The manager responds that Beulah does not get release time from work for the visits, and since the clinic hours correspond with her work hours, she may not keep all her appointments on that basis. She adds that Beulah probably is worried about the salary loss even though the treatments are paid for, seeing that she is the sole breadwinner for herself, her disabled husband, and two small grandchildren. The manager says she will talk to Beulah about the unacceptability of her failing to let the Occupational Therapy Department know when she decides not to keep her appointment. In fact, if Beulah keeps that up, the manager says, she will find herself paying for the missed appointments, since the hotel can't be expected to pay for her lack of responsibility. Tiffany responds that maybe Beulah didn't know about the policy. The manager replies, "It doesn't matter. She knows better than that. By the way, she has been here at the times you mentioned, so at least she wasn't off on a shopping trip or anything like that."

A week goes by. At the scheduled time for Beulah's appointment, she does not appear. Tiffany has been uneasy about the conversation with the manager, and when the time comes for her to fill out the billing slip for another missed appointment, she feels positively terrible.

Just to help you prepare for the discussion, take a minute to make a few notations about the following:

In this narrative, what are some missing parts that would help you better evaluate the situation? For example, what details of their stories (Beulah Watson's, Tiffany Bryant's, and the hotel manager's) would help you to have greater certainty about the ethical problem Tiffany is facing? Write them here.

_____

_____

_____

Do you share Tiffany's feelings that something just is not right? Yes _____
No _____

If yes, what do you think is the problem or problems?

_____

_____

_____

What type of person would you want to be if you were in Tiffany's shoes?

_____

_____

_____

What do you think Tiffany should do? Why?

_____

_____

_____

In answering these questions you have used key ideas already presented in this book: the ways in which narrative is relevant to ethics, the importance of character traits, and the duties, rights, consequences, and principles that you can call upon when deciding a course of action. All three are necessary if you are to begin applying your knowledge and skills to actual ethical problems.

COMMON COMPONENTS OF THE THREE PROTOTYPES

The three prototypes of ethical problems involve one or more of the following components:

A—a moral *a*gent
C—a *c*ourse of action
O—a desired *o*utcome

We will take each in turn.

A—The Moral Agent

What do you think an agent is?

In ethics or law an agent is anyone in a situation in which she or he is responsible for the outcome of her or his actions. Obviously, agency requires that a person be able to understand the situation and be free to act voluntarily on her or his best judgment. It also implies that the person intends for something to happen as a result of that action. A *moral agent* is

> [A]ny being who is capable of thinking, deciding and acting in accordance with moral standards and rules. A moral agent may not always fulfill the requirements of a moral standard or rule, that is, he need not be morally perfect. But he must have the capacity to judge himself on the basis of such a criterion and to use it as a guide to his choice and conduct.[2]

In the preceding story there are at least three moral agents, Tiffany, Beulah, and the hotel manager. This book emphasizes *your* role as a moral agent in the health profession setting since at the very least you can answer for your own actions and attitudes.

C—The Course of Action

The course of action includes the agent's judgment process and decision. As we discussed in Chapter 1, applied ethics uses the concepts and tools of ethics to deal with practical ethical problems that arise in a specific situation. In the story above, Tiffany Bryant used the information she had and made the call to the hotel manager. This could well have arisen from a sense of moral responsibility she felt not to continue to bill the company for treatments Beulah did not receive. Afterward, her discomfort may have meant that she was not sure she had exercised the correct moral judgment in making the call to the hotel manager.

O—The Desired Outcome

The desired outcome is the hoped-for result(s) of having taken a particular course of action. We are not sure what Tiffany was hoping would happen when she called the hotel manager.

Having acquainted yourself with the components of ethical problems, you are ready to explore the three prototypes.

ETHICAL DISTRESS: BARRIERS TO AGENCY

Type A   Type B

A ——————————//—————— O   or   A ——————————//—————— O
     C Certainty   C Uncertainty

Ethical distress focuses on the agent (A) herself or himself. When you are the agent, ethical distress denotes the psychological discomfort you feel when you are blocked from being the kind of person you want to be or from doing what is right. Agents encounter two types of barriers: type A and type B.

Type A: There Is a Barrier Keeping You from Doing What You Know Is Right

To illustrate this, Jameton uses the plight of nurses at one institution who know the right thing to do but for whom it is nearly impossible to pursue the right course of action because of institutional constraints, a situation that could apply to other health professionals as well. For example, a hospital may routinely give all entering patients an unnecessary battery of blood tests. This costly practice imposes unnecessary risks on patients and is therefore an unethical practice. But staff nurses employed by the hospital have neither the personal authority nor access to the decision-making channels needed to change the practice. Moreover, it is personally risky for staff to criticize a practice that helps the hospital make ends meet.[3] Here the right course of action (C) leading to the desired outcome (O) may involve the nurses' talking to the patients to expose the unethical practice or talking with the laboratory people to try to influence the unethical policy. The ethical distress comes precisely because of the repercussions the nurses believe they would have to endure. There are institutional and traditional role barriers keeping them from exercising their agency for the good of their patients.[4]

Type B: There Is a Barrier Because Something Is Wrong, but You Are Not Sure What It Is

The barrier may not be policies or practices but instead may be the fact that the situation is new or extremely complex. Your only certainty is an acknowledgment that something is wrong; the rest is a big question mark. You may question the morally correct course of action (C) or what to work toward as a desired outcome (O). The challenge is to remove the barrier of doubt or uncertainty by further analyzing the problem, using all the tools of ethical analysis available to you.

You can see that the psychological response of ethical distress is the first sign to most health professionals that something has gone—or is about to go—wrong, something that will threaten you or your profession's integrity. *Integrity* comes from the Latin for "fittingness" or "wholeness." A threat to integrity arises when you cannot be the person you know you should be in your professional role. The internal signals are warning you there is something wrong: a knot in the pit of your stomach, a catch in your easy stride, waking up in the early hours of the morning with the haunting feeling that something is awry. As you learned in Chapter 2, emotions, feelings, and experience are critical data of the moral life, and now they are trying to work for you to say, "Stop! Wait! Don't! Think twice!"

But you also will need character traits, discussed in Chapter 3, as resources in this situation: your compassion, caring, commitment to competence, courage. The virtues act as motivaters, goading you to correct some-

thing you know is wrong or to increase your certainty about the right decision to make.

Think about Tiffany Bryant. She feels uneasy. I asked you to think about
why you might feel uneasy too if you were in her situation. I assume that her
discomfort partially stems from her wanting to do what is best for Beulah
Watson but not being sure she has. She wants to be a compassionate and
caring health professional, but she is not sure she is. Understandably she also
wants to honor the rules and policies of her workplace but is not sure she
should be charging for Beulah's missed treatments. Her ethical distress is
more of type B, as I read her situation. What do you think?

_____

_____

_____

Tiffany's task as a moral agent in this situation is to continue to reflect on
and analyze the situation. (In Chapter 5 you will learn a step-by-step
method for analysis related to ethical conduct.) As she reflects, Tiffany
thinks about whether her distress is related to the fact that she is facing an
ethical dilemma. So that you might join her in that reflection, we turn to the
prototypical ethical problem, ethical dilemmas.

ETHICAL DILEMMA: TWO COURSES DIVERGING

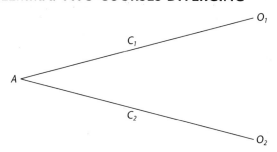

Many people call all ethics problems ethical dilemmas. More correctly,
an *ethical dilemma* is a common type of problem that involves two (or more)
morally correct courses of action that cannot both be followed; that is, to
take course C_1 precludes you from taking course C_2. As a result you (the
agent, the responsible one) necessarily are doing something right and also
wrong (by not doing the other thing that is also right). You are between a
rock and a hard place, between the devil and the deep blue sea.

Sometimes ethical dilemmas involve conflicting traits of character. If
you think it is best to be honest with patients but you have now encountered
a situation in which to be honest with the person may cause her great dis-

tress, even to the point of discontinuing her work with you, you have a dilemma. Your honesty and your compassion have presented themselves in a situation where you can exercise one option but only at the expense of the other.

More often, ethical dilemmas involve ethical conduct. As you may remember from your reading of Chapter 3, the conduct-related theories of ethics are the deontological (with the emphasis being on duties and rights), the utilitarian (with its emphasis on consequences), and the use of principles as guides.

Suppose that Tiffany Bryant has just read the above paragraph and realizes that before she called the hotel manager she had an ethical dilemma but did not recognize it at the time. She was aware of her ethical distress and that further analysis was needed. Here is why she now knows she had a dilemma:

On the one hand, Tiffany is an agent (A) who has a duty to respect her patient, Beulah Watson, and in Tiffany's role as health professional, the course of action (C_1) that will express that respect is in the form of giving Beulah the treatment that is best for her. The desired outcome (O_1) is the relief of the patient's pain and stiffness. The element of ethics Tiffany uses for her reflection on her duty to Beulah Watson is beneficence. On the other hand, Tiffany is an agent (A) who has a duty to abide by the policies of her place of employment. The course of action (C_2) that will express her loyalty is to charge for all treatments that are given or are not officially canceled. The desired outcome (O_2) is the financial solvency of the occupational therapy clinic as well as a recognition that patients have a responsibility to show up for their scheduled appointments. The element of ethics Tiffany uses for her reflection on her commitment to be a good employee is fidelity. Both outcomes are ethically appropriate, taken alone. However, Tiffany Bryant probably caused some negative repercussions for the patient. Therefore she maintained fidelity at the price of beneficence.

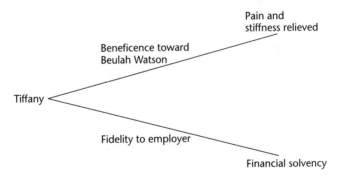

Of course, Tiffany might have thought that charging for missed appointments is wrong under any circumstance, a position being examined in the health profession literature because this practice is increasing in health care institutions.[5]

I have been guiding you to think primarily in the mode of ethical elements or principles because most health professionals' ethical decisions are made by weighing such considerations (whether or not the agent uses the technical language of principles). Our oaths and codes rely on principles. This approach is consistent with deontology because principles often are viewed as duties or rights. If you were analyzing this as a utilitarian, however, the _____ would be the focus of your analysis. You would be weighing the good brought about by O_1 (i.e., Beulah's pain and stiffness symptoms are relieved) against that brought about by O_2 (i.e., the financial solvency of the department). You may find other consequences to put into the equation.

To further apply what you have learned, I will ask you to go back to the story of Ron Rachels (Chapter 2). What is his ethical dilemma?

If you said that Ron believes Pamela Faden's right to autonomy involves her right to know about the mistake so that she can decide what to do about it *but* that Ron also has a duty not to harm her in the form of undermining her trust in Dr. Kristansen, you have correctly identified one plausible way of thinking about his ethical dilemma. Schematically it looks like this:

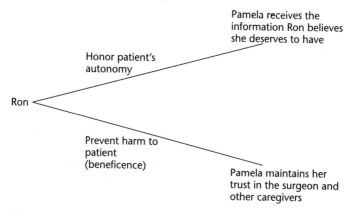

Each course of action Ron contemplates is ethically correct according to the principles of autonomy and beneficence. But to act on one necessarily will compromise the other.

The Special Case of Paternalism

Sometimes an ethical dilemma presents itself in this manner: The patient's autonomy, or choice, conflicts with the health professional's judgment of what is best for the patient based on the professional's values, which are not necessarily those of the patient. In other words, the conflict is between the patient's choice and the professional's judgment of what is best for the patient. This type of dilemma is called a situation of *paternalism* or *parentalism*.

The word itself suggests that the health professional is acting as a _____. If you answered *father* (from paternalistic) or *parent*, you have grasped the concept. This is such an important idea that you will have an opportunity to think about it in several of the stories that follow. In fact, in subsequent chapters you will have an ample opportunity to work with several types of dilemmas because it is a commonly confronted type of ethical problem.

The Special Case of Distributive Justice

Another special ethical dilemma arises in regard to allocating societal benefits and burdens justly. As in all ethical problems the agent (A) makes a judgment to take a course of action (C) that results in an outcome (O). The situation is this: competition exists for a cherished but scarce resource such as medication, health professionals' time, money to pay for health care, or an organ or other types of life-saving procedures. The agent's (A) morally right course of action (C) is to give everyone a full measure of the resource to the extent he needs or merits it. In so doing, the outcome (O) will be that the patients' legitimate claims were honored. The scarce supply, however, requires that the agent take difficult, even tragic, courses of action, the outcome being that some claimants will get the cherished good and others will not. In short, it is morally right to give your own patient everything he needs to benefit from your interventions, and it is also morally right to distribute the resources justly. You cannot do both.

Can you think of an example of how you might become involved in this type of dilemma? If so, write it here:

_____

_____

_____

LOCUS OF AUTHORITY PROBLEM

A *locus of authority problem* raises the question of who should have the authority to make an important moral decision. In other words, the question is, Who is the rightful agent (A) to carry out the course of action (C) and to decide the desired outcomes or results (O)?

I think of this as a "second level" ethical problem because it is not about the type of person you, the agent, should be or the type of action you should take. Therefore it does not fit tidily into the usual categories of ethics re-

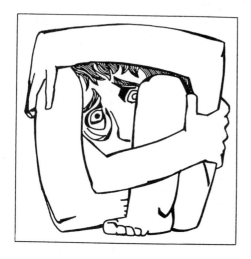

FIGURE 4-1 Facing ethical problems. From Purtilo, R., and Haddad, A. 1996. *Health Professional and Patient Interaction*, 5th ed. Philadelphia: W.B. Saunders, p. 21.

garding moral character, duties, rights, or principles. Still, in Chapter 2 we discussed the importance of *context* in ethical decision making. It does matter who has decision-making power in institutions. For instance, if you work in a situation in which one person or group *always* has the say-so because of a degree after her name or because of a title he holds, then you know the ethical distress that led you to further ethical reflection is coming from the fact that you have no agency. Figure 4–1 illustrates how health professionals who are *not* in a position to act responsibly sometimes feel.

Locus of authority problems most often arise when roles or other institutional policy or societal arrangements create *ambiguities* about who is in charge. Schematically the problem looks like this:

$$A_1 \underset{C_1}{\rule{3cm}{0.4pt}} O_1 \quad \text{vs} \quad A_2 \underset{C_2}{\rule{3cm}{0.4pt}} O_2$$

Note that two people assume themselves to be agents (A_1 and A_2) and proceed along different courses of action (C_1 and C_2). Logically they may come to different conclusions about how to achieve the best outcome (O_1 vs O_2) for a patient. In the story of Tiffany Bryant and Beulah Watson, who do you think should make the decisions about whether to charge for missed treatments?

- The health professional providing the service _____
- The supervisor of the unit _____
- The institutional administrator _____
- The government or some other, larger societal regulating body _____

Sometimes there is no ambiguity, but reflection on the issue reveals that the wrong person is the one with the authority. The challenge of determining the appropriate locus of authority is the topic of thoughtful reflection by ethicists and others. In the health professions context, there are at least four ways of thinking about authority in health care decisions:

1. *Professional Expertise.* You are in a professional role along with other people in different professional roles. This is the essence of teamwork that characterizes so much of health care today. The role differences mean that you bring different spheres of expertise to the situation. In some areas of the patient's care each is *an authority* about some part of the whole picture. That, alone, should be a vote for the person who has the most relevant knowledge about the patient's condition and other factors to be the decision maker.

2. *Traditional Arrangements.* Traditionally in the health care system the physician has been the authoritative voice in health care decisions by virtue of his or her role as a physician. In other words, the physician is considered *in authority* because of his or her office or position rather than (or in addition to) being *an authority* because of special expertise. From this perspective the medical director of the unit would unquestionably be the one to make a decision about what to do, although he or she may choose to invite advice and counsel from other persons.

3. *Institutional Arrangements and Mechanisms.* Sometimes the decision about the authoritative voice will come from special institutional arrangements. For example, some tasks may be delegated to committees. In these instances the committees or designated individuals assume specific task-related roles. This is really a variation of the first two, the designated persons being *in* authority both because of expertise and the position he or she holds. For example, it is possible that the authority for making a decision regarding billing for missed treatments may be referred to a committee designed to deal with humane treatment of patients in unusual situations rather than treating billing solely as a finance issue.

4. *The Authority of Experience.* Occasionally a voice of authority will emerge because of the insight that comes from experience. There are always those situations in which we seek the advice of people who have been in similarly perplexing situations and defer to their judgment. Tiffany Bryant may wish to seek advice for the next step from a supervisor, senior member of the professional staff, or other person judged to have the benefit of experience. This is seldom institutionalized as a formal mechanism for dealing with locus of authority problems and is a variation of the professional expertise approach, which assumes that expertise often is refined with experience in a wide range of situations.

SUMMARY

This completes your introduction to the basic prototypes of ethical problems that will confront you in the several roles you may assume as clinician, administrator, researcher, teacher, and team member.

Questions for Thought and Discussion

1. Jane is a medical student who does not want to treat an AIDS patient in the intensive care unit because she is afraid of contracting AIDS herself. Her supervisor assures her that she is safe as long as she uses the universal precautions designed to make the treatment of persons with infectious diseases safe for everyone. Jane still hesitates saying, "I know it's irrational, but I'm afraid I will not be effective because I'm so scared." Using the three prototypes of ethical problems you have learned, what type of ethical problem do you think Jane has?

2. Find a newspaper or magazine article this week that portrays an ethical problem and analyze it using the schema presented in this chapter.

3. Describe an ethical dilemma that has faced you or someone you know. This does not have to be a problem that arose within the health care context.

References

1. Mann, T. 1927. *The Magic Mountain* (H.T. Lowe Porter, Trans.). New York: Alfred A. Knopf.
2. Taylor, P.W. 1975. *Principles of Ethics: An Introduction*. Encino, CA: Dickinson Publishing Co.
3. Jameton, A. 1984. *Nursing Practice: The Ethical Issues*. Englewood Cliffs, NJ: Prentice Hall, p. 6.
4. Jameton, A. 1993. Dilemmas of moral distress. AWHONN *Clinical Issues in Perinatal and Women's Health Nursing* 4(4):542–551.
5. Fay, A. 1995. Ethical implications of charging for missed sessions. *Psychological Reports* 77:1251–1259.

5

A Six-Step Process of Ethical Decision Making for You to Follow

Objectives

The student should be able to:
- Identify six steps that will help professionals analyze and, when possible, resolve ethical problems encountered in everyday professional life.
- List four areas of inquiry that will be useful in trying to gather relevant information about a situation.
- Describe the role of imagination in arriving at practical alternatives.
- Discuss how will, integrity, and courage are factors in being able to take action.
- Describe two benefits of taking time to reflect on and evaluate the action afterward.

New Terms and Ideas You Will Encounter in This Chapter

Physical restraints
Chemical restraints

Topics in This Chapter Introduced in Earlier Chapters

TOPIC	INTRODUCED IN	DISCUSSED IN THIS CHAPTER ON
The importance of story or narrative	Chapter 2	Page 82
Ethical distress	Chapter 4	Page 84
Ethical dilemma	Chapter 4	Pages 84–85
Locus of authority problem	Chapter 4	Pages 85–86

Introduction

You have come a long way in laying the foundation for identifying prototypes of ethical issues and problems. In this chapter you will have an opportunity to apply what you have learned and to use a problem-solving method to analyze and resolve problems. The story of Anthony Carnavello and Alex Myers is a good starting point for this discussion.

THE STORY OF ANTHONY CARNAVELLO AND ALEX MYERS

Alex Myers, a social worker, has just begun working in a municipal nursing home. The facility has a reputation for maintaining high standards of care. When Alex was interviewed for the position, he made a thorough tour of the home and talked with several employees and residents. Everything seemed "in order," and he took the job.

It is now near the end of his second week of work. Alex goes to the nursing home office to read the personal record of a resident who may be transferred to another facility because of his apparent worsening mental status. He learns that Mr. Anthony Carnavello is 76 years old and has diabetes. Recently his left leg was amputated because of complications from a fracture of his left femur sustained in an accident. According to the record he fell in the corridor of the nursing home after tripping over a chair. Reportedly he is "confused" most of the time and is kept quite heavily sedated "to keep him from becoming violent." He is almost blind. There is no neurological report in the record.

Alex decides to introduce himself to Mr. Carnavello before going to lunch. When he finds Mr. Carnavello's room he is surprised to see a shriveled-up little old man lying in bed staring at the ceiling. Alex introduces himself and tells Mr. Carnavello that he will be coming back to visit with him in the afternoon.

Mr. Carnavello squints in an effort to see Alex. Abruptly he raises up on one elbow and says, "I'm so scared! They keep giving me shots and pills that make me crazy! Can you get them to stop?"

Just then a nurse comes into the room with a syringe on a tray. "Anthony!" she says in a firm, loud voice. "Turn over on your side, please. It's time for your shot!"

Mr. Carnavello protests that the pills and shots are making him "crazy as a hoot owl." But the nurse has exposed one loose-skinned buttock and is deftly injecting the solution before Mr. Carnavello succeeds in resisting. He tries to take a swipe at her, but she backs off quickly. She pats his bony hip, saying, "There now, you're OK, Tony," and leaves immediately. Mr. Carnavello lies back on the pillow and sighs. He grabs the rail, pulls himself up toward Alex, and says, "See what I mean!" Alex thinks that Mr. Carnavello looks genuinely anguished. He reaches out to pat Mr. Carnavello's hand, but Mr. Carnavello pulls it away and falls back against the sheet.

Alex is angry and confused. There is a gnawing feeling in his stomach that something is wrong in the way Mr. Carnavello is being treated. At lunch he shares his concern with Annette Carroll, the nursing supervisor for the entire home. She is highly respected by residents and staff alike. He tells her it seems to him that Mr. Carnavello is not being treated with the dignity that the residents deserve. He doubts that Mr. Carnavello is "violent" but can't put his finger on why he felt so much anger at the nurse who efficiently and without undue harshness gave him the injection. Maybe it is because he believes the medication is being used to "dope" Mr. Carnavello unnecessarily. As he recounts what happened, he can feel a seething rage rising up in him. He decides, on the spot, that he will talk to the nursing home administrator and announces that intention to Ms. Carroll.

She listens attentively. When Alex pauses for a few disinterested bites of his sandwich, she says, "Alex, you have been here only two weeks. I can understand your uneasiness at what you thought you saw happening. And maybe you are right—maybe Mr. Carnavello is not being treated with the respect he deserves. But remember, being new here, there is much that you don't know. We are doing for him what we think is best as well as trying to protect our staff from his dangerously aggressive behavior. He was worse before we started him on Haldol."

Alex doesn't feel any better after lunch. He'd like to talk to someone and decides to call a social worker who works in another nursing home.

As in most actual situations, Alex's first encounter with what appears to be an ethical problem has left many questions unanswered. The path from Alex's first perception to possible action traverses a six-step process.

THE SIX-STEP PROCESS

Ethical analysis requires your thoughtful reflection and logical judgment even though the situation usually presents itself in a mumbo jumbo of partial facts and strong reactions. The following steps allow you to take the situation apart and look at it in a more organized, coolheaded way while still acknowledging the intense emotions everyone may be experiencing about the situation.

In Chapter 1 you learned that when everyday morality requires you to pause and reflect, you engage in ethical reflection. Ethics is reflection on and analysis of morality. Therefore this step-by-step process is, overall, a formalized approach to reflection.

Step 1. Get the Story Straight: Gather Relevant Information

The first step in informed decision making is to gather as much information as possible. Anyone viewing this situation might ask the following types of questions:

- Does Mr. Carnavello have organic brain disease that might explain his behavior?
- What tests have been conducted to confirm the type and degree of brain involvement?
- What does his "violent" behavior consist of?
- What might have happened in Mr. Carnavello's history to make him afraid of the nursing staff or the whole setting and, therefore, to react in a hostile manner?
- Has the Medical Director been made aware of Mr. Carnavello's complaints about the effects of the medication?
- What is the recent history of the exchanges between this person and the staff?
- What other approaches (besides medication) to Mr. Carnavello's ostensibly violent behavior have been—or could be—attempted?
- What evidence is there that approaching the nursing home administration will create problems for Alex, Ms. Carroll, or others?
- What other information about physical and chemical restraints in nursing homes should Alex seek out?
- Are there other questions you thought of as you read the story?

The necessity for close attention to details takes you back to Chapter 2, where you were introduced to the importance of the story or narrative. Without knowing as much as possible about the story line it is impossible to ascertain the moral values and duties embedded in it. The fact-finding mission is absolutely essential as a safeguard against setting off on a false course from the very beginning.

Some of the benefits of seeking out the facts in the situation described above are that you may be able to determine whether Alex's perception of Mr. Carnavello's treatment is accurate and to understand why the various players in this drama are acting as they are. Although Annette Carroll's comments are difficult to interpret, she may be implying that Alex's response would be tempered by more knowledge of the situation. Often what initially appears to be a "wrong" act is, after all, a right or acceptable one once more of the story is known.

Fact finding could also help Alex identify the focus of his anger more specifically. What triggered the response? Was it Mr. Carnavello's apparent helplessness in the situation? The nurse's actions? What he has read about chemical restraints and the OBRA '87 regulations?[1-3] Why Mr. Carnavello has been labeled as "confused" and "violent" when he showed no signs of being either?

The work of Jonsen, Siegler, and Winslade offers four major areas of inquiry regarding "facts" that may be useful to health professionals who are trying to gather the relevant information about any situation.[4] You should learn to refer to them as a mental checklist during your data gathering and add specific questions in each area appropriate to the specific situation.

1. *Clinical Indications*
   a. What is the diagnosis or prognosis?
   b. Is the illness or condition reversible?
   c. Is life-saving treatment medically futile?
   d. What is the present treatment regimen?
   e. What is the usual and customary treatment for this type of condition?
   f. What is needed to relieve suffering, provide comfort?
   g. Who are the primary caregivers?
   h. What can you learn about this person's medical history?
2. *Preference of the Person*
   a. What does he or she want in this situation?
   b. Who has communicated the realistic options to the person?
   c. What was the person actually told?
   d. What evidence do you have that what the person said has been heard by key decision makers?
   e. Is she or he competent to make decisions about this situation?*
   f. If not competent, does the person have a living will, advance directive, or other document indicating her or his considered preferences?*
   g. Is another person speaking as a legitimate surrogate for this person?*
3. *Quality of Life*
   a. What are the person's beliefs and values about what matters in life? (This will require that you go back to item 2 above, since the only appropriate judge of this question is the person herself or himself.)
   b. What quality of life considerations are the decision makers bringing to this situation, and how are their biases influencing the decision processes?
   c. Is there any hope for improvement in the person's quality of life?
4. *Contextual Factors*
   a. What institutional policies may influence what can be done?
   b. What are the legal implications (court cases, statutes, etc.) regarding this issue?
   c. Are scarce resources an issue?
   d. How will these services be paid for?

---

*These issues are discussed in more detail in Chapters 11 and 12.

When you have searched out the information you and others deem relevant or are convinced no additional helpful information will be forthcoming, you are ready to proceed to the next step.

Step 2. Identify the Type of Ethical Problem

Even while his initial fact finding is taking place, Alex can begin to *determine the type of ethical problem (or problems)* he is facing. You know that in the beginning his worry was something like this:

> Mr. Carnavello is a human being. Human beings always should be treated with dignity. Part of being treated with dignity includes allowing a person to take part in his or her own treatment decisions whenever possible and in Mr. Carnavello's case includes at the very least being treated with sensitivity to the anguish that he appears to be experiencing. To ignore his distress shows a lack of compassion, if not outright cruelty, and reduces him to the status of an object. I think that Mr. Carnavello is not being treated as a person ought to be treated.

This is where the prototypes of ethical problems you encountered in Chapter 4 begin to work for you.

Ethical Distress

You know that Alex is experiencing *distress*. He has witnessed a scene that baffled him, and he finds himself not able to forget about it. My guess about the fundamental basis of Alex's distress is his perception that Mr. Carnavello is not being treated with the dignity he deserves as a human being. The distress, then, arises from Alex's role as a professional with a moral responsibility to help uphold human dignity. In other words, he is an agent in a situation that he surmises involves morality and that, because it is worrying him, merits his further attention. As he puts more information in place, he may confirm that his distress is, in fact, *ethical distress type B*. (For a quick review, see pp. 70–72.) You can also presume that he is a caring, compassionate person. Otherwise he would not be worried about what he witnessed.

Ethical Dilemma

Goaded by his character traits and the awareness that he is experiencing ethical distress, he will be better able to decide whether he also has an ethical dilemma (or dilemmas).

> Alex learns that quite a few of the staff (but not all) believe the medications are being used disproportionately to the amount of "violence" Mr. Carnavello has been demonstrating. In fact, some of the staff confide that they believe he is being sedated to keep him more in line with the conduct of the other more docile and cooperative residents. Of course, the nursing home is shorthanded,

and the administrator makes this point when Alex finally goes to talk with her. Her argument is that if everyone took as much time and extra attention as Mr. Carnavello does (when unmedicated), no one would receive a fair amount of treatment. Mr. Carnavello also seemed very agitated and suspicious at times, and the medication has helped to improve his feeling of security. Finally, she mentions that some of the staff are afraid of Mr. Carnavello, and she has a responsibility for their safety too.

There are several issues here that Alex, as an employee and team member, may be implicated in as partial agent. Foremost of these is whether they, as a team, are acting ethically in the use of restraints under any circumstances. The one ethical dilemma that falls squarely on Alex's shoulders at the moment, however, looks like this:

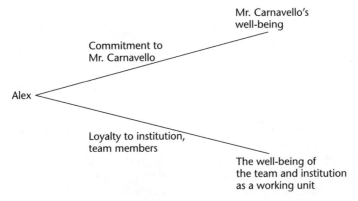

His dilemma arises from the fact that Alex has become more persuaded that he was right about what he saw happening to Mr. Carnavello but also that he can agree with the points made by the administration and some of the staff regarding Mr. Carnavello's relative comfort, the fairness to other residents, and the idea that Alex is only one member of a team that needs to work harmoniously in order for Mr. Carnavello (or any other resident) to be well taken care of. He is experiencing difficulty in deciding what to do. In short, he has an ethical dilemma.

Locus of Authority Problem

If Alex decides someone other than himself, the administration, or the team should be making decisions regarding any aspects of Mr. Carnavello's treatment (or the nursing home policies regarding treatment), he also faces a locus of authority ethical problem. For instance, although the story does not give you the benefit of knowing whether Mr. Carnavello's input is being included in the decision, Alex could decide that the authority for this decision should rest with Mr. Carnavello. From what we have been told we can assume that the staff and medical director have determined that he is not competent to make such a decision and that therefore they are acting paternalistically. The question that Alex is struggling with on one horn of his dilemma is whether the medications truly are being given with Mr. Carnavello's benefit in mind.

Step 3. Use Ethics Theories or Approaches to Analyze the Problem(s)

In Chapters 2 and 3 you were introduced to normative ethical theory and approaches. In Chapter 4 you learned that situations requiring the health professional to be an agent (i.e., take action for which she or he is morally accountable) draws on ethical theories that focus on duties and rights or consequences. In other words they are the conduct-related theories. It may help jog your memory to take this short matching quiz:

1. Utilitarianism focuses on the overall _____.   A. means

2. Utilitarianism is a particular type of _____   B. consequences
theory.   C. teleology

3. Deontology focuses on _____.   D. duty*

4. Deonto (Gr) means _____.

Alex's story may make it easier to compare the two theories than when they were presented in the abstract.

If agent (A), Alex, is like most health professionals guided by the principles of duty and rights in his professional role, he probably will decide that his weightier (i.e., more compelling) responsibility is to Mr. Carnavello. He will be acting according to the principle of beneficence.

If agent (A), Alex, approaches it from a utilitarian standpoint, he will spend less time thinking about his duties or the principles of ethics and will be guided by his desire to bring about the overall best consequences in this situation. The overall best consequences may be to "leave well enough alone," not to make waves with the nursing home administrator or others.

Which approach do you find yourself leaning toward in this situation? Why?_____

_____

Step 4. Explore the Practical Alternatives

Alex has decided what he *should* do. The next step is to determine what he *can* do in this situation. He must exercise his imagination and confer with his colleagues regarding the actual strategies and options open to him. Sup-

---

*Correct answers: 1. B; 2. C; 3. A; 4. D.

pose he decides that his initial perceptions were correct and that he must act on behalf of Mr. Carnavello, even though the staff sees no problem.

At this juncture many people oversimplify the range of options available to them. They tend to fall back on old alternatives when under stress, a behavioral pattern you can probably recognize from your own stressful situations. Therefore, imaginative pursuit of options is a big challenge—but an invaluable resource—in resolving ethical problems. In recounting Alex's story we learned that he believed his range of options was to confront the nursing home administrator or do nothing. A diligent search for other options can now make the difference between his doing the right thing and allowing a moral wrong to go unchecked.

Applying your own imagination to his situation, list all the alternatives you believe Alex has. Try to identify at least four:

1. _____

_____

2. _____

_____

3. _____

_____

4. _____

_____

Having listed them, which one do you think is the best? Why?

_____

_____

_____

Often it is a good idea to try out some of the more far-fetched alternatives with a colleague whom you trust and with whom you can share the situation without breaching the patient's confidentiality. Alex did this with the nursing supervisor. We do not know how her counsel helped him in the end, but we are sure that her words led him to further examination of what his next step should be.

Step 5. Complete the Action

Think of all the work Alex has already done: He responded to his initial feeling that something was wrong, followed his compassionate disposition that motivated him not to let the matter go unnoticed, reasoned about and decided upon the type of ethical problem(s) he was encountering, carried out an analysis using one or more of the ethical theories and approaches, and exercised his imagination to identify practical options. He also shared his worry with at least one other person he knew commands the respect of others and himself. Now he has one more task, but it is the crucial one, and that is *to act*.

If Alex fails to go ahead and act, the entire process so far will be reduced to the level of an interesting but inconsequential philosophical exercise or, worse, may result in harm to Mr. Carnavello. Of course, Alex may consciously decide not to pursue the situation any further, but insofar as it involved his deliberate intent, it is different than simply failing to follow what seems a correct course of action. If harm comes to Mr. Carnavello or others because of Alex's inaction or unnecessarily narrow focus, he will be an agent of harm by his own omission or neglect. The solid ethical foundation he laid in steps 1 to 4 will have been of no use.

Why would anyone fail to act in this type of circumstance? Mainly because it is sobering to be an agent in such important matters of meaning and value in others' lives. Some decisions are literally life and death decisions; all are of deep significance to the people facing the particular situation. Although the previous step required imagination, this final step requires the strength of will to go ahead, knowing there may be risks or backlashes. As Alex becomes more experienced he will be increasingly aware that his will and purpose must be supported by his compassion, integrity, and courage.

Step 6. Evaluate the Process and Outcome

Once he has acted, it behooves Alex to pause and engage in a careful *retrospective* examination of the situation. The practical goal of ethics is to resolve ethical problems, thereby upholding important moral values and duties. The extent to which Alex's decision led to action that upheld morality, however, is knowable only by reexamining what happened in the actual situation.

This evaluation is germane to his growth and development as an ethical professional and is essential if the outcome he hoped for was not realized. In the clinical setting a widespread mechanism for addressing interventions that go awry is morbidity and mortality (m and m) rounds.* The m and m rounds allow health professionals whose interventions did not yield the hoped for results to present the case to their peers for further evaluation. Sometimes ethical committees or your own unit staff meetings con-

---

*If you have not yet been in the clinical setting the term *rounds* may be new to you. Rounds is the general term used for meetings of clinicians. Some are held sitting in a room (sit-down rounds), and others are held walking from patient to patient (walking rounds).

duct *ethics* morbidity and mortality rounds to have a group review of a particularly difficult situation that seemed not to yield the hoped-for ethical outcome.

Suppose you, like Alex, have just been through the process of arriving at a difficult ethical decision and have acted on it. Some questions you might ask yourself are the following: What did you do well? Why do you think so? What were the most challenging aspects of this situation? How did this situation compare with others you have encountered or read about? To which other kinds of situations will your experience with this one apply? In answering the preceding two questions you are doing the work of casuistry introduced in Chapter 2. Who was the most help? What do the patient, family, or others have to say about your course of action? Overall, what did you learn?

SUMMARY

If you studied this chapter carefully you will have identified the following six-step process that anyone faced with an ethical problem can use:

1. Gather as much relevant information as possible to get your facts straight.
2. Determine the precise nature of the ethical problem (if the data confirm that there is one).
3. Decide on the ethics approach that will best get at the heart of the problem.
4. Decide what should be done and how it best can be done (explore the widest range of options possible).
5. Act!
6. Reflect on and evaluate the action.

Questions for Thought and Discussion

1. The first step in ethical decision making is to gather as much relevant information as possible.

   The information-gathering process, however, can become so extensive that it becomes an end in itself and could actually deter one from proceeding to action at all. What types of guidelines would you use to decide that you have as much information as you need or can obtain?

2. A necessary step in ethical decision making is to act on one's own conclusions about what ought to be done. Under what conditions, if any, would you decide **not** to act according to your own best moral insights and judgment? That is, what, if any, are the limits to your willingness to act ethically?

3. In your professional practice you would much prefer always to act ethically. What type of supports or assurances within your work setting would enable you to so act?

References

1. Fletcher, K. 1996. Use of restraints in the elderly. AACN *Clinical Issues* 7(4): 611–635.
2. Farrell-Miller, M. 1997. Physically aggressive resident behavior during hygienic care. *Journal of Gerontological Nursing* 23(5):24–35.
3. *Omnibus Budget Reconciliation Act PL100-203 (1987) Subtitle C. Nursing Home Reform.* 1987. Washington, DC: United States Government Printing Office.
4. Jonsen, A., Siegler, M., Winslade, W. 1998. *Clinical Ethics: A Practical Approach* (2nd ed.). New York: Macmillan, pp. 6–25.

Ethical Dimensions of Professional Roles

6

Surviving Student Life Ethically

Objectives

The student should be able to:
- Describe some barriers to ethical decision making peculiar to the student role.
- Identify six areas where students have full moral agency in the professional practice setting.
- Discuss two types of wrongdoing students may encounter and what should be done in each case.
- Assess the availability and usefulness of policies, procedures, and practices designed to enhance students' ethical development and decision making.

New Terms and Ideas You Will Encounter in This Chapter

Legal fraud

Topics in This Chapter Introduced in Earlier Chapters

TOPIC	INTRODUCED IN	DISCUSSED IN THIS CHAPTER ON
Postmodernism	Chapter 2	Page 96
Ethical distress	Chapter 4	Pages 96, 97
Type A		
Type B		
Role of emotion	Chapter 2	Page 97
Ethical dilemma	Chapter 4	Pages 97, 98
Utilitarianism	Chapter 3	Page 98
Ethical elements, principles	Chapter 3	Page 98
Veracity (truth telling)	Chapter 3	Page 98
Beneficence	Chapter 3	Page 98

Introduction

The ethics foundation presented in Section One will serve you well during your student days as well as throughout your life. This chapter and the next focus on your personal moral development and the need to exercise ethical decision making throughout your career, beginning with the time you are a student. It is especially important to include your role as student and some of the particular opportunities and stresses of this period because no matter your age, the student years are the time your approach to ethical decision making in your professional role takes shape.

SPECIAL CHALLENGES OF STUDENT LIFE

As a student you have the advantage of coming into a situation with a fresh perspective and can raise issues that more seasoned professionals would miss or might gloss over. At the same time, a situation sometimes is misjudged solely because students do not have the advantage of having served in a professional role or in a particular setting for a long time.[1]

The story in this chapter highlights some ethical challenges inherent in your role as a student.

THE STORY OF MATT AND THE BOTCHED HOME VISIT

Matt Weddle is a nursing student in his next to last year of professional education. He has enjoyed his professional training and especially enjoys being in the actual patient care environment. Today, however, he went to bed discouraged and wondering if he has made the correct career choice.

Matt is on a home health care rotation. He has an excellent supervisor, Ms Needleman, who has tried to provide him with a wide range of learning experiences and proper supervision during his time with her. This has not been an easy task: the census for the home care association is high, and with major cutbacks in professional staff she has been busier than usual. He is sorry to learn that she is going on vacation tomorrow and that his supervision will be turned over to Mr. Cripke, another nurse.

Today Ms Needleman asks Matt if he would stop by Mrs. Bedachek's apartment to check on her son and be sure his wound is healing well. "If necessary, the wound may need debridement and a bandage change. You can make the judgment about whether to change the bandage, since I changed it myself yesterday on my way home from work." He is somewhat uncomfortable about going alone to see a patient he has not seen before. He also remembers being told by his academic clinical coordinator at school that under no circumstances should he go into a patient's home unsupervised. But he agrees to do so, not feeling free to question Ms Needleman about whether this is correct procedure. Instead, he assures her that he has done this procedure enough times under her supervision that he feels he should be able to do it. She agrees.

When he knocks at the Bedacheks' door a large woman in a filthy housedress peers through a crack in the door. At first she doesn't want to let him in, but when he shows her his name tag as identification that he is "the nurse," she admits him. He introduces himself with his name and says he is a student nurse. Mrs. Bedachek is already walking laboriously across the room toward the other occupant, an equally large mentally retarded man. The man strains to peer at Matt from a large armchair set up in the midst of the clutter in the small living room. Matt knows the man's name is Tom, but he is unprepared for the greasy-skinned person drooling onto the front of a mucus-stained shirt.

When Matt tells the patient what he has come to do, the man grunts. The woman says, "I don't want you to touch that bandage. It's fine." She draws up the man's shirt for Matt to see. Matt is surprised at the size of it and concerned about the dark seepage around the bottom edge. Mrs. Bedachek says, suspiciously, "Who are you again?" Matt repeats his name. "At least you're not a student," she says. "They're the worst." Matt says nothing. He feels uncomfortable about this whole situation. He reaches toward the bandage to touch it, and she suddenly pulls the shirt back down over her son's trunk. The stench is making Matt feel woozy.

"Really, it's fine," she says.

Matt replies, "OK," and leaves.

When he gets back to the office, Ms Needleman is there, clearing off her desk. "How did it go?" she asks. "Fine," he says. "Well, you did wonders. I didn't want to tell you, but most people can't get through the front door. I went myself yesterday. I thought the wound looked really good except for that distal edge."

Matt had meant to tell her immediately about the whole scene, but for some reason her comments unnerve him and he feels like a failure. He says, "Yeah, I agree."

She comes over to him. "Thanks so much for getting me through that squeeze. I knew you could handle that bandage change, and I was worried about letting it go." She continues, "Sometimes I think it's not worth trying to go on vacation!" She pauses and extends her hand, saying "I have enjoyed working with you as a student. You will make a fine nurse. And you will enjoy working with Mr. Cripke."

She leaves hurriedly, saying she has to pick up her son at daycare and get packed. Matt takes Tom Bedachek's record from the drawer and writes, "Wound debridement, bandage change. Purulent exudate around the distal rim of wound."

Almost everyone would agree that both Ms Needleman and Matt Weddle exercised poor judgment. As you look at the story through Matt's eyes, what do you think are the reasons he is feeling discomfort after the day's events?

_____

_____

_____

As a student you do not always know the best thing to do, and there may be psychological and structural barriers to your acting on what you think is right. What type of ethical problem is this? _____

_____

If you answered "ethical distress," you are remembering well what you have learned. As soon as you begin your on-site education in the setting where you will pursue your professional career, the opportunities to use this type of ethics knowledge present themselves. With that in mind you have an opportunity in the next few pages to walk in Matt's shoes and explore the ethical implications of his situation.

USING WHAT YOU HAVE LEARNED AND ACKNOWLEDGING STUDENT LIMITATIONS

You already have learned a lot about the analysis of ethical issues. Let us go over some of the ways in which this fits the ethical distress prototype.

One of the barriers to Matt's doing the right thing is that he does not feel at liberty to question his supervisor's request to go to the Bedachek's home alone and, apparently, also does not feel able to tell her the truth after his botched visit. Ms Needleman has not presented the situation in such a way that he has reason to fear her disfavor: She does not appear to be motivated to wield her power unfairly or to be punitive. Also, nothing we know about Matt leads us to believe he is devious, lazy, or dishonest. In fact, his anxiety and subsequent behavior may be at least partially explained by the nature of the student-teacher relationship in which the imbalance of power between the two is built into the structure. Matt's situation is an example of why some of the approaches you encountered in Chapter 2 (e.g., some postmodernist approaches) place so much stress on imbalances of power within institutional structures themselves. This would fit the _prototype of ethical distress type A_ in which there is a structural barrier to Matt's doing what his better moral judgment would dictate.

He also may be experiencing _ethical distress type B_. He knows a lot but is still in training. Understandably there are unknowns related to the limited professional experience Matt brings to the setting. He knows how to change a bandage and to debride a wound. But the larger *narrative* of the story leaves many gaps for him to fill in as he goes along. For instance, perhaps he has had limited experience talking with people like the Bedacheks. He may never have seen a person with the degree of mental impairment Tom Bedachek manifests. He is not sure how to instill enough confidence in either of them to figure out how to get on with the wound debridement. He also is being forced to reckon with his new realization that in home care a professional is a stranger who is invading the private lives of people and that adaptation to their home environment is essential to successful intervention.[2]

In Chapter 2 you studied about the role of emotion in ethical decision making. Matt is frustrated, afraid, angry. His being overwhelmed by the enormity of the unknown and his being insecure in his judgment about what to do are not unusual student responses. As a student yourself you may recognize a tendency to discredit your own feelings, intuitions, and judgments. The worst outcome of this student-related stress is that you may assume you are completely unable to evaluate a situation correctly or even to get enough information to make a sound judgment about it. The best outcome is an enhanced awareness that you deserve help: the student years are the time to become as well prepared as possible, and good teachers should assume you will need a lot of assistance. In other words, your emotional responses can be a positive sign of something that needs attention.

In short, I propose that his situation fits the prototypes of type A and B ethical distress. Do you agree with my analysis? Why or why not? What have I missed?

_____

_____

_____

Let us continue to analyze Matt's problem, considering whether he also has an *ethical dilemma*. If so, this is your opportunity to describe it.

_____

_____

_____

I suggest he may have faced more than one dilemma! One that seems directly related to his student nurse status arose around Mrs. Bedachek's comment about how students are "the worst." When Matt first introduced himself, he identified himself as a student nurse. We do not know his motivation for remaining silent when she made the derogatory comment about students. He had an opportunity then to reaffirm his student status, which definitely would have been the right thing to do. Let us give him the benefit of the doubt, however, and assume that his reason for remaining silent was that he truly believed this was the only way he could hold on to the little bit of confidence Mrs. Bedachek had in him and that he had to allow this deceit to benefit Tom Bedachek. You have had some experience now in schematizing ethical dilemmas. Sketch out this one as I have described it. The basic framework is presented:

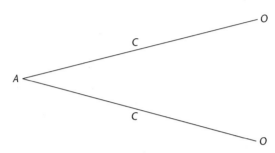

Sometimes patients are less comfortable with students than with others, so Matt's judgment to remain silent as a way to allow the patient the benefit of feeling comfortable is consistent with his duty of beneficence. Of course, the motivation might also be to bolster his own confidence, which is not, in itself, a bad thing. If you are reasoning about this as a *utilitarian*, you are on the path to legitimating this course of action on the basis of the overall good consequences you believe will result. Within professional ethics, however, the commitment to truth telling is vital as a means to maintaining the patient's confidence or trust. Using the principle of *veracity*, Matt cannot easily justify withholding such key information without believing that he is engaged in wrongdoing. He may decide to forgo veracity to honor his duty of beneficence, but believing he has compromised an important ethical principle, he cannot comfortably carry out his course of action. As you might recall, an ethical dilemma creates the type of difficult decision in which you have to allow something wrong to happen (i.e., in his case, to withhold the truth from her) while you are also allowing something right to happen (i.e., being able to provide needed treatment to her son Tom). This clearly illustrates how the student role does not protect you from ethical dilemmas you will have to face on your own. During your formative years as a student the sixth step of the decision-making process you learned in Chapter 5 (Evaluate and reflect on the decision) is important in helping you refine your ethics skills.

TAKING RESPONSIBILITY

You have already learned (see Chapter 4) that for a person to be held morally responsible for her or his actions the person must be the moral *agent* in the situation. In your student role you may have had to sign a student honor code. Many universities have such honor codes and other ethical guidelines detailing the range and scope of your moral agency and accountability generally (e.g., must refrain from plagiarism, other types of cheating and deceit, use of illegal substances, disrespecting others). The topic becomes more complex in professional educational programs in which moral responsibilities related to your role as a student professional are added. For example, an analysis of Matt Weddle's story reveals there were times he felt he was in a position to take full responsibility for his choices and others when he knew he was not the agent or was not sure if he was. Some factors in his variable degrees of agency are the nature of his role as a student, the character of the student-professor relationship, and his inexperience regarding some life situations in general.

Fortunately the degree of agency you have as a student professional is not totally ambiguous or random. You have a moral responsibility to:

1. Take full advantage of your student role to refine your ethical decision making under supervision.

Most of Matt's experience was characterized by this type of situation. Until their last day together Ms Needleman gave him ample opportunity to practice his skills under her supervision in a variety of settings. He had the benefit of continual discourse and feedback from her. By actually taking the opportunities seriously he was acting responsibly by learning as much as he possibly could before having to make such decisions on his own. Only when she asked him to do something without her supervision did he run into difficulty. Once you graduate you will no longer have the formal ethical and legal protection to make poor judgments that you have as a student.

2. Express serious doubts about your qualifications to your supervisor if you have been given the authority by that person to act independently.

In retrospect you can see that Ms Needleman used poor judgment in sending Matt to the Bedachek's home alone. Even though she thought he was capable of completing the technical procedures competently and independently, she had not thought through all the ramifications of the situation he might encounter. For instance, she was not being responsive to the literature that warns how important the availability of colleague consultants is in the home care treatment environment.[3] It was her moral responsibility to do so, especially in her role as supervisor, and in that respect she failed to exercise it well. In fact, if Matt's actions (or in this case, failure to act) led to litigation against the caregivers, she would have been held legally responsible for what "her" student did or did not do.

That does not leave Matt Weddle in a position of having no moral responsibility, however. His moral agency extends to the point of his telling her he has doubts about his capabilities. This is true even though there are all the reasons we discussed for his ethical distress. In fact, it is his knowledge that he *can*—has the capacity to—express his hesitance that makes it appropriate to characterize him as the moral agent in an ethical distress situation. Likely this awareness is also one of the reasons he feels so disquieted at the end of the day.

3. Refrain from acts that would be wrong for anyone to commit.

This situation includes morally wrong or illegal acts that are not specific to your role responsibilities as a student professional. These are actions for which you would be held equally accountable as a citizen. It also includes refraining from the exercise of immoral character traits that would be harmful in any relationship in which someone trusted you to treat him or her fairly and with respect.

What is an example of Matt's failure to exercise his moral agency and take responsibility for his actions that would have been the same in any relationship?

_____

_____

_____

You may have found several places where you think this happened. I assume you agree that one occasion was his deceit by silence and lying. The more glaring example of this was his decision to report on Tom Bedachek's record that he had performed the therapeutic procedure when he had not. His deceitfulness and dishonesty are not tied to the health professional and patient relationship: intentional lying is harmful to the moral values and duties that help bond us as a community. The principle of _____ is the name given to this type of ethical element. (If you have forgotten, look back at the list of principles outlined in the list on page 50.) There seemed to be no circumstance that would excuse him from this important principle of morality. Making himself look more responsible than he was could not justify his lying.

Entering false statements on a medical record is also illegal. He is committing _legal fraud_ because the home health care agency will be paid for treatment it did not perform. This act could cost him his professional career and lead to criminal sanctions as well. What are some of the reasons this breach of professional responsibility is viewed as so serious by society as a whole?

_____

_____

_____

4. Share what you know when the effectiveness of the health care team depends on information you have about the patient and other aspects of the situation.

Matt Weddle knows how Mrs. Bedachek feels about students. He knows how hard it may be for anyone to come into the Bedachek home and be able to do what they have come to do for Tom. That fact alone could be critical information for the home health care team as they plan their schedules. During this one visit, what other information did Tom gain for the future that you would consider relevant to good patient care?

_____

_____

_____

Sometimes students are great reservoirs of information. Although I mentioned previously that patients or clients may be hesitant to let students treat them, the converse often is true too. Some patients feel safe in telling a student things they do not want to say to professionals:

> Sometimes the empathic student is a patient's most articulate and effective advocate, energetically protesting what he may construe as negligence, indifference, or just plain wrong-headedness by . . . [health professionals]. Clearly the eager interest, constant questioning, and active participation by students greatly enhance the effort, attention and application of staff.[4]

In such moments you are a key member of the team in regard to planning optimal treatment approaches.

5. Be ready to help identify the best alternatives possible for patients, or clients, and others who are faced with difficult situations.

One of the reasons health professionals enjoy working with students is that students often provide creative approaches to old problems. Professionals who have been facing similar issues for years get bogged down in habit or become discouraged because attempted solutions have not been successful in the past. (How many times have you heard, "We've tried that before, and it didn't work"?)

I suggest that your unwillingness to offer suggestions is not a morally neutral act. Sheer robustness, arrogance, or ill-placed criticisms are not welcome. At the same time, your moral agency as a student extends to voicing your thoughtful opinion when you are invited to do so and taking a posture of readiness to contribute such ideas rather than standing by passively and keeping your insights to yourself.

Although Matt has breached some moral guidelines in his moral agency in the student role, he can still offer suggestions from the perspective of what he observed at the Bedacheks. Of course, he also has a moral responsibility to contribute his thoughtful ideas regarding all the other situations he has had the opportunity to witness and participate in during his tenure in this clinical setting.

6. Remain faithful to your own convictions and exercise the will and courage to voice them.

Abstaining from Wrongdoing

Some general protections for health professionals to avoid moral compromise were introduced in Chapter 1. Similar protections should apply to students. For instance, during your student experience you have a moral responsibility to make your convictions known so that you are never placed under pressure to participate in a procedure that undermines your religious or other deeply held convictions. Religious observances may pose another reason for you or your fellow students to want special consideration, say, to participate in holiday traditions and rituals. Every professional educational program should have a formal or informal mechanism in place to assure that you and your student colleagues are able to offer rationales for wishing to abstain and to have an appeals process in place for disagreements. Of course, you have the responsibility to inform your educational program administrators and supervisors in advance of any such situation so that patient care is never compromised. Whenever possible there should be plenty of lead-in time for your request to be heard and considered in a timely manner.

Righting Wrongdoing You Have Committed

Another dimension of living according to your convictions is to right any wrongs you yourself have done. No one enjoys having to do damage control after wrongdoing, but there is no better investment than taking care of yourself by keeping your conscience clear. Practice during your student years is critical if you are going to be able to admit shortcomings and mistakes throughout your career. When approached thoughtfully, professors and supervisors almost always are forgiving and stand ready to discuss and help prevent such breaches from happening again.

Matt should admit his wrongdoing of lying about the wound dressing as soon as possible. If you were Matt, how would you go about correcting this terrible error in moral judgment?

_____

_____

_____

What would you hope for in terms of a response from your supervisor?

_____

_____

_____

Addressing Others' Wrongdoing Constructively

This arduous moral task is also a part of everyone's responsibility in the health care environment, including yourself and your fellow students.

Quiet, diligent observation is a reliable guidepost in your assessment of wrongdoing by your fellow students or by professionals. A legitimate worry about expressing your concern arises because as a student you often do not have full knowledge of the situation. We noted in the last chapter that Alex Myers, who had completed his social work preparation and was an employee, hesitated after talking to Ms Carroll because she warned him that he did not "have all the facts." To make fact-finding more confounding, as a student you are not an actual employee of the institution in which you are placed and therefore are unfamiliar with its policies. Finally you probably do not know the in-house mechanisms employees use for resolving concerns and conflict, and even if you do, they may not apply to you.

In the end these information-gathering challenges should not keep you from addressing ethical problems. For instance, Matt probably does not need any more information to know with certainty that Ms Needleman acted wrongly in sending him to the Bedachek's home alone, no matter her rationale.

The first step in the six-step process of ethical decision making is to gather relevant information, and the preceding caution is a reminder that as a student you must be extra vigilant and is not to be taken as a suggestion that you not act on what you know for certain.

A more thorough, step-by-step description of the decision-making process applied to reporting wrongdoing among colleagues is addressed in Chapter 8. The steps are similar whether you are a student or full professional, and therefore it is appropriate to wait until then to go into more detail. A final comment on the student's special challenge in regard to the six-step process arises around step 4, explore the practical alternatives. You are advised to use the channels set up for students in your professional program. Your clinical supervisor and academic supervisor are two obvious places to begin. Most educational programs have institutional policies and procedures to protect students who follow the processes designed to protect the legal rights of everyone involved while encouraging responsible reporting of wrongdoing.

If you have run into this situation, jot it down here so that you can refer to it as you proceed through this book. Perhaps you will gain some ideas regarding how you could have dealt with it effectively.

I was troubled when I saw or heard the following:_____

_____

_____

_____

At the time I handled it by _____

_____

_____

_____

I think this was an effective _____ not so effective _____ way to handle this problem. Ideas I have now for how it might have been handled better:

_____

_____

_____

There are plenty of reasons students never pass the test of exercising their moral agency by following up on others' wrongdoing. One is the fear of reprisal. The student who "makes waves" sometimes fears becoming the target of reproach from those who themselves are not beyond reproach. In some situations this fear is realistic, although, when the cautions outlined above are followed, it is rare. Another reason for ignoring the problem is the awareness that you will be "moving on." It is easy to rationalize away the responsibility by thinking the temporary nature of your position as a student in the setting makes you less culpable than the employees. Neither will serve you well in the long (and sometimes the short) run: There will never be a time in your professional career when you will be free of such fears and rationalizations, so putting off accepting responsibility does not prepare you better for what is ahead. If you fail to act in clearly defined ethical dilemmas, you will be creating a habit of neglect and withdrawal that can only worsen as your responsibilities increase.

SUMMARY

In summary, there are special ethical challenges during your student role that involve both the peculiarities of the student-supervisor or professor relationship and the limits of your own knowledge and experience. At the same time, the story of Matt Weddle's experience in the Bedachek's home illustrates several ways you may exercise your moral agency and be accountable for what you have done. It is the mutual task of students, classroom faculty, and clinical supervisors to ensure that students trust their abilities, understand their role as moral agents, and act appropriately. In fact, the purpose of this book is to help you think clearly about a wide variety of ethical situations before you are faced with the more weighty responsibilities associated with professional practice following completion of your studies.

Questions for Thought and Discussion

1. Peter is in his final year as a student in the clinic. For some reason this particular internship setting has been full of rough edges. Peter and his supervisor have just never really hit it off, but when he talked to his academic coordinator about his feelings, the coordinator urged Peter to "keep trying." Moreover, the coordinator claimed that the supervisor thought Peter was "doing great." When his final evaluation came, it was barely passing. For Peter the most disturbing comment on the report was that he has an "attitude problem." He believes it must be because he reported his problems to his academic coordinator, whom he has always trusted. Now he feels betrayed and alone.

   Does Peter have an ethical problem? If so, what is it? What should he do in this situation? What are the moral responsibilities of each of the people involved?

2. This morning Andrea, a student working in the outpatient clinic, notices two men sitting in the waiting area. She recognizes one as her dad's business partner, Mr. Brown, and greets him. She recalls that in a recent visit she made to her parents' home for dinner her father had expressed concern about Mr. Brown's failing health, which has begun to interfere with his earnings. Mr. Brown and the other man are chatting amiably in spite of the fact that they make a striking contrast—the silver-haired Mr. Brown and the seamy young man with a torn leather jacket. She remembers her dad's admiration for Mr. Brown's ability to "cross classes" and have friends in all walks of life.

   Andrea is somewhat shy about her assignment to take Mr. Brown's medical history, but does not feel at liberty to tell her clinical supervisor. Mr. Brown seems relaxed about it, however, and even a little bemused as she earnestly questions him and checks off the answers on her sheet. She leads him into the next room to prepare him for his tests, and on the way something falls from his pocket. In a moment of curious uncertainty she does not call it to his attention. Once he is in the dressing room, she rushes back and picks up the packet. Inside the brown bag is a syringe and a small plastic bag of white powder. On the outside, written in a smudged scrawl on a piece of white tape, it says, "Brown, $450." She feels panic rising up in her chest and hopes beyond hope that her suspicion is unfounded.

   If you were in Andrea's situation, what do you believe you should do or not do? Does her role as a student professional dictate what she should do in regard to sharing this information with her father? That is, would it make any difference if she had met Mr. Brown on the street and her terrible discovery had been made?

   Discuss the steps you would take in arriving at your decision, emphasizing the professional moral duties, rights, and character traits that will help to inform and guide your decision, as well as the special challenges you face as a student professional in this setting.

3. You overhear a fellow student say to another colleague, "I just pretended to treat her. She was sleeping and will never know the difference anyway. It's such a drag to have to treat someone who's out of it."

   a. What breaches of professional ethics are apparent? What should you do, and why?

   b. This student has cheated a patient out of her treatment. How is this different from cheating on a classroom test? If you observed classroom cheating, should your response to it be different than it would be to your knowledge that the patient was not treated?

4. You have learned in your preclinical professional education that use of a certain procedure has been discontinued almost everywhere because of a dangerously high incidence of harmful side effects. You observe it being performed regularly in the setting where you are presently assigned, a place with a good reputation (apparently well deserved, generally speaking). In fact, as you observe patients' responses to the procedure, you become convinced yourself of good reasons *not* to use it. Now you have only one week left in this rotation and raise your concern with your supervisor. She responds, "Actually, we know that, and we don't like it either. Our health plan, however, does not allow us to use the newer procedure because it is four times as expensive as this one."

   Do you have a moral responsibility to recommend this site be discontinued for students? Why or why not? Do you have a moral responsibility to do anything in this situation?

5. Your friend who is serving in the same clinical setting with you stops you in the hallway to ask you what he should do. His wife has called, crying, saying she feels really sick and would like him to come home right away. He has already missed several days because his uncle died, and he also had a bout of the flu. The supervisor spoke with your friend this morning about how they would have to try to make up for some of the absences by providing special opportunities for him to cover areas he has missed. In fact, she told him that she has arranged for him to assist in an evaluation that starts at noon and will take about four hours but from which he will benefit tremendously. He cannot get home and back in time for the beginning of the procedure.

   How should you respond? Why? _____

   _____

   What do you think he should do? Why?_____

   _____

6. This chapter focuses on your *clinical* education experiences. What are some ethical problems that students may face in the *classroom* during their professional preparation? Discuss one, utilizing the tools you have acquired from your study of ethics so far.

References

1. Purtilo, R., Haddad, A. 1996. *Health Professional and Patient Interaction*, 5th ed. Philadelphia: W.B. Saunders, pp. 69–83.
2. May, B.J. 1993. *Home Health and Rehabilitation*. Philadelphia: F.A. Davis.
3. Collins, J., Bessner, K.I., Krout, K. 1998. Home health physical therapy: Practice patterns in western New York. *P.T. Magazine* 78(2):170–179.
4. Bradley, S.E. 1978. The medical student as moral agent. *Bulletin of the New York Academy of Medicine* 54(7):646.

7

Surviving Professional Life Ethically

Objectives

The student should be able to:

- Evaluate the phrase "you owe it to yourself" from the standpoints of a duty to be good to yourself, aspirations for yourself, and responsibility to yourself.
- Identify two key responsibilities to yourself that help health professionals lead a good life.
- Describe three components of a personal values system and its relationship to personal integrity.
- Evaluate your own personal values system.
- Identify two types of challenges to personal integrity encountered in the health professions and some strategies for meeting them successfully.
- Define self-deception and identify five types of self-deception that can challenge your personal integrity.
- Describe two societal mechanisms designed to legally protect health professionals faced with professional situations that would undermine their personal integrity.
- Identify three types of responsibility to improve yourself that are relevant to your professional career.

New Terms and Ideas You Will Encounter in This Chapter

A duty to be good to yourself
Duty of general obligation
Duty of special obligation
Aspirations regarding
   self-fulfillment

Responsibilities to yourself
Personal values system
Personal integrity
Self-deception
Impairment

Topics in This Chapter Introduced in Earlier Chapters

Topic	Introduced In	Discussed In This Chapter On
Duties	Chapter 3	Page 110
Integrity	Chapter 4	Page 113
Cooperation with wrongdoing	Chapters 1 and 6	Page 110
The principle of material cooperation	Chapter 1	Page 110

Introduction

You have come a long way in thinking about the ethical dimensions of professional practice in a general way, and in Chapter 6 you focused on them in relation to your role as a student. This chapter gives you an opportunity to think about loyalty to yourself as you assume your professional role and throughout your professional life.

JANICE K AND THE POLICIES OF HER WORKPLACE

Janice K. is a dietitian employed by a community health clinic affiliated with a large multihospital health plan. Part of the mission of the clinic is to provide nutritional counseling and services for people in an underserved area. She believes that part of her professional responsibility is to help assure that people in such areas have access to health care benefits like everyone else, and she is delighted to have found this position. Janice is distressed, however, when she learns one day that the health plan has designated her clinic as a site where abortion counseling and services will be added to its family planning programs. Janice has strong religious convictions that abortion is murder and that this practice should be stopped by whatever means possible.

Janice is trying to decide what to do. She has been talking with her religious advisors, friends, and colleagues about her feelings, all of whom were well aware of her position before the announcement. They have different ideas about what her response should be. Among the suggestions she has received are the following:

1. Distribute antiabortion pamphlets around the clinic.
2. Talk with clients in the clinic to get their opinion and be guided by their needs.
3. Quit working in a place like this and find another job.
4. Pray about this turn of events.
5. Call some groups who will come and picket the clinic in protest.
6. Talk to the administrator of the clinic and try to persuade those in authority not to include this service.

7. Tolerate the situation—it is a pluralistic, diverse society, and some people will want to take advantage of the abortion service who could not receive it elsewhere.
8. Go about her work diligently and not get involved in taking care of any of the abortion patients.

This story could lead to many interesting and important ethical discussions, but in this chapter we will focus on the prime importance of your personal morality as the ethical wellspring of survival in your professional career. You have had some opportunities to think about your personal values and personal morality already in the course of reading this book: In Chapter 1 you were introduced to the idea of cooperation with wrongdoing, the principle of material cooperation being used as a guide, and some ways in which society tries to protect professionals. In Chapter 6 personal morality was raised again in regard to areas where you must exercise your moral agency as a student. So far every story in this text has posed an ethical problem to you as you try to put yourself into the shoes of the person who is the moral agent. Now you have an opportunity to step back and focus on yourself directly.

In this chapter, Janice is confronted with an ethical challenge, and you can try to help her think through her strategies. You read what other people advised her to do. What do you believe she should do?

_____

_____

_____

I asked you, What do you *believe* she should do? not solely, What do you *think* she should do? because any answer you provide will involve your analysis of **her** values and of **your** beliefs as well!

Her beliefs are powerful sources of what Janice thinks her duties and character should be. You too owe it to yourself to try to live by your beliefs.

YOU OWE IT TO YOURSELF

How does one operationalize this odd phrase, "You owe it to yourself"? Does this mean that you have *a duty to be good to yourself* to live by your values? In Chapter 3 duties were placed under the umbrella of society's expectations of moral conduct between individuals or social institutions. They describe commitments persons should make to *other people* to act in certain ways that are believed to uphold the moral life of the community. Ethical theorists often delineate duties more fully in the language of the specific principles or elements you were introduced to in Chapter 3. And so it is unusual to talk about a duty to *yourself*, although I will give you an example of one philosopher who has done so. W.D. Ross, a British philosopher writing in the early 1900s, was influential in developing the idea of moral obligation, and he included the "duty of self-improvement" among his list of duties. He believed that the duties of beneficence (toward others) and *self-improvement* arise because we should produce as much good as possible. He called both beneficence and self-improvement *general obligations* in contrast to special obligations. *Special obligations*, he said, arise from the special relationship in which we stand to each other (e.g., parent-child, professional-patient or client; teacher-student) and include nonmaleficence, fidelity, gratitude, and reparation, to name some. General obligations rely less on specific relationships. In other words, Ross treated self-improvement as making sense as a duty in that it brings about good generally, but, of course, you are the major beneficiary![1] In short the idea of a duty to oneself seems awkward to most ethical theorists, but Ross contributed to our understanding of the moral life by reminding us that we should have a strong commitment to ourselves as well as others if our search for moral excellence is to succeed.

Another way to think about the idea of owing it to yourself is less related to duty and more to giving yourself permission to rejoice in having achieved an aspiration. An *aspiration* is an ideal standard of excellence toward which you strive, and when you have attained that standard you have gained a point toward your self-fulfillment. Anytime you realize such an aspiration, you deserve (i.e., owe it to yourself) to reward yourself. For example, when you have aspired to lose weight or make a high grade in a course and you achieve it, you may owe it to yourself to acknowledge your success by going out to buy a new pair of jeans or taking time from studying to read a novel. Similarly, in the realm of the moral life you may aspire to be courageous, to go the second mile, or to set an example of high moral character for others. Has there been a time recently when you experienced this kind of self-satisfaction? The primary reward in this case is in seeing the good you are capable of bringing about and knowing you have made a stride in developing a high moral character. You owe it to yourself to enjoy the good it has done for others. You owe it to yourself to be aware that next time it will be easier. You owe it to yourself also to reward yourself with writing it here and taking some time to remember it before reading on.

_____

_____

_____

Yet a third way of conceptualizing what it means to owe something to yourself is to think of *responsibilities to yourself*. Responsibility includes accountability but also has the root idea of responsiveness embedded in it.[2] In other words, it has the force of commitment that the language of duty captures, but it also entails the idea of responding to your aspirations to live according to your personal ideals. I find this notion of responsibility to yourself the richest way to understand that we owe something to ourselves insofar as it places a claim on us to act in certain ways that will benefit us and gives us permission to celebrate that we have developed the moral character disposing us to do so. The following discussions introduce you to two responsibilities to yourself that will serve you well throughout your professional career, the responsibility to *maintain personal integrity* and the responsibility to *engage in self-improvement* as a person.

THE RESPONSIBILITY TO MAINTAIN PERSONAL INTEGRITY

You have been concentrating on your responsibility to think clearly about complex ethical situations before acting. Part of the way to achieve this skill is to learn about and honor the duties, rights, and character traits required in your professional role. But here is the rub: As the cases so far have clearly illustrated, these helpful approaches to analyzing professional conduct sometimes come into conflict, and an ethical problem arises. Just as a review, what are the three prototypes of ethical problems?

1. _____

2. _____

3. _____

If you cannot remember, go back to Chapter 4 to review them.

When one of these problems arises, you must call on your own *personal values system* to help you decide what to do.

What *is* a personal values system? A personal values system is the set of values you have when you have reflected on and chosen values that will help you lead a good life. Usually people adopt personal values that partially overlap with societal values and that are in harmony with them. Elsewhere I have represented and explained them in more detail according to the following scheme[3]:

PERSONAL VALUES SYSTEM

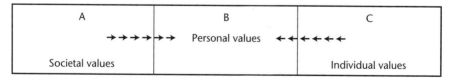

A	B	C
→ → → → → →	Personal values ← ← ← ← ← ←	
Societal values		Individual values

Area A represents values developed by society. Many times we accept these values because we want to live easily and harmoniously in society. Examples include obedience to traffic laws or other laws, adherence to etiquette, and willingness to pay taxes. Area C represents individual values that are important to you simply because you value them individually. You receive personal benefits from them. The area of overlap, area B, represents values that you have internalized so that they not only are shared by other people in society but also are perceived as your own values. The motivations for accepting them are that leading a good life includes not only living harmoniously in society but also experiencing personal satisfactions and self-fulfillment. For many, some of these values include friendship, economic independence, and the realization of certain character traits such as fairness or courage. Most people integrate these three into a lifestyle and personal values system, drawing at times on all three areas, A, B, and C.

This personal values system provides the components whereby your actions can be guided by a sense of personal integrity. *Integrity* comes from the Latin *integritas*, meaning unimpaired, sound, whole, a sense of fittingness. It can be applied to both individuals and groups. The goal of integrity is to enable you to act on your own convictions in a meaningful way for your own life. At the same time, it acknowledges that at times conflicting ideas must be brought together in a whole. The conflicting ideas for Janice K. are (1) continuing to work in a setting that provides abortion services when she believes that abortion is wrong, (2) refusing to work there, or (3) disrupting the center's functioning in an act of protest.

In Chapter 1 you listed some values that are important to you. Take a few minutes to reflect on them and try to put them into the larger context of your personal values system:

_____

_____

_____

Opportunities to Strengthen Your Personal Integrity

At least two major forces may challenge your personal integrity. At the same time, they present opportunities for professionals to examine and further strengthen their personal value system by taking advantage of how new information sometimes can lead to refinements of personal insights. Each is addresssed in turn, with strategies for strengthening your resolve to lead a good life guided by your highest values.

The Challenge of "Bad" Laws, Policies, and Regulations

Personal integrity can be challenged by *bad laws, policies, or regulations*. These might be poorly stated, so that they provide poor guidance, or, worse, might be morally wrong in their emphasis. In Janice's situation the center's general policy of providing access to persons in underserved areas is consistent with her personal values system and convictions. Only when the abortion services are added does this new policy become a threat to Janice's personal integrity. She has done the wise thing in seeking the counsel of her friends, colleagues, and others in thinking about this threat, although she undoubtedly has encountered differences of opinion. She wants to know what her role should be in trying to maintain her personal convictions in the face of this new policy.

One factor that will influence her decision is her sense of personal integrity that requires her to try to work within the system to bring about alternative policies she believes best serve the population they are designed to serve. Another is her judgment about what of value will be lost if she actually leaves. A third factor is her assessment of whether there is any way she can indeed influence the administration to change the policy. To come to a decision she will have to consider the priorities in her own values system. She may need to write down her priorities and let her actions be guided by those that have top priority.

Moving beyond Janice's story you can think more broadly about this idea of how policies and regulations can challenge your integrity. Every health professional should read the play *The Dark at the Top of the Stairs*, by the great American playwright William Inge, because it is a fine illustration of how persons sometimes are unwilling or unable to interact with the "powers that be" who make and revise policies. The setting for the play is the home of the Rubin Flood family in a small Oklahoma town, where he, his wife Cora, and their two children are living. It takes place in the 1920s, during a prosperous time for this area because of an oil boom. What we see of the Flood's house is the living room, but there is a flight of stairs at one side, and at the top of it is a second floor landing. Some of the most vital activity in the play, the moments that set direction for the rest of it, are played out on that landing, but the Flood family never integrates those activities into the process of resolving the small sorrows, tragedies, and missed opportunities that finally threaten their integrity as individuals and as a family.[3]

This family's story holds a lesson for health professionals. Many policies that cause consternation because they appear to challenge one's personal integrity can be challenged and changed. Awareness of the important value of maintaining personal integrity should provide an opportunity for cooperative effort aimed at changing such policies even though maintaining your integrity may mean getting involved with the higher-ups. Can you think of a health care policy that would present such an opportunity to strengthen your personal integrity? If so, jot it down here.

_____

_____

_____

Before leaving this topic I want to add that an opportunity to examine the specific components that make up your personal integrity may come from your self-perception of your professional role and what is required in it. For example, if Janice perceives her role as a dietitian as being one that has no place in changing policies not directly related to dietetics, she will feel more vulnerable and may believe that her only option is to leave. At the same time, if she discerns that a part of her role generally is to question policies in her workplace that threaten her personal integrity, she will feel more empowered to act within the system. In the latter case she must be prepared to present her ideas to the people who are involved in making and revising the family planning policies, understanding that her beliefs and convictions may not prevail in the final outcome. At the very least she will know she has made an effort to stop a practice that she thinks is morally wrong. By being willing to speak her mind within the system, she may also have an opportunity to hear the arguments on the other side and learn the reasons why other people are supporting them even if she is not persuaded to support them herself.

The Challenge of Self-Deception

Self-deception can also pose a challenge to your personal integrity, although it has nothing to do with policies or the perception of your role in an institution.

Self-deception is engaged in by all of us at one time or another. The Christian scriptural text instructs, "Do not try to remove the moat in another's eye until you have removed the beam from your own."[4] The Russian novelist Gogol observed, "Do not blame the looking glass if your face is awry." Unfortunately sometimes a challenge to personal integrity comes from within, the result of engaging in self-deception about what is best for yourself or others. When a person's self-esteem is threatened, he or she may resort to the extreme measure of self-deception to try to protect himself or herself. This, of course, backfires. In his book *Morality and Self Deception*, Martin provides the following paradigm of self-deception:

1. **Willful ignorance** . . . absence of true belief.
2. **Systematically ignoring** . . . distraction of unpleasant thoughts to more pleasant ones.
3. **Emotional detachment** . . . protection of self-esteem by detaching oneself emotionally.
4. **Self-pretense** . . . a struggle to believe that something is not true.
5. **Rationalization** . . . belief that one's own view is necessary whether substantiated or not.[5]

In short, self-deception is blindness to self-acknowledgment. "To thine own self be true" or "Know thyself" is an old adage attributed to Aristotle. The obligation to know ourselves is threatened by our need to protect a faltering self-esteem by evading what we really know.

Self-deception should be treated as a form of *impairment*. Institutions have methods for dealing with impairment that include team conferences and support groups, in-house counseling and education for dealing with uncertainty. Because self-deception hides the need for this type of help from the person who needs it, input from a caring colleague or supervisor usually is required for the problem to be addressed. Offering insight and support to your colleagues and employees in these situations can help the development of their as well as your own moral character.

Societal Safeguards Revisited

Near the end of Chapter 1 you were introduced to several ways moral compromise of your values can be minimized by safeguards that society provides for persons in their professional role. Now that you have examined how personal integrity is at the root of your ability to survive ethically in your professional role, it is fitting to review the societal safeguards briefly.

First, in situations in which the courts become involved, one of the state's interests is to protect the *integrity of the professions*. For instance, in one case, Elizabeth Bouvia, a young woman with cerebral palsy, asked not to be fed in the hospital so that she could die there. Many of her health professionals said, "Morally speaking we cannot do this; she will starve to death, and it will be our fault." The case was taken to court, and the courts upheld the health professionals' point of view, partly on the basis that the personal integrity of the professionals would be threatened by performing this act.[6]

Additionally, abstaining on the basis that you find a procedure "morally repugnant" may be allowed if you can show why you believe it will threaten your personal integrity to participate. This idea was developed when abortion first became legalized in the United States because it was known that some professionals would judge the procedure to be morally wrong.

Both these lines of reasoning could be used by Janice K. She would not be personally involved in performing the abortion procedure, but she could argue on behalf of her physician and nurse colleagues who are afraid they will be directly involved in having to participate in abortions. The rich interplay of society and an individual in the professional role continues to work itself out through such laws. Fortunately the cherished value of personal integrity is not overlooked in society's understanding of what you should or should not be required to do.

Personal Integrity and Personal Vigilance

In this chapter the difficult and often heated subject of abortion is used as an illustration of how some persons' integrity may be challenged. The question of how to maintain personal integrity arises in many more subtle situations as well. The autonomy and elevated status of being a professional, along with society's willingness to protect you from participating in activities you believe are wrong, provides safeguards for you so that you can maintain personal integrity in the practice of your profession.

At the same time, societal safeguards cannot identify the content of your beliefs and values. You are the only one who can maintain the vigilance necessary to treat your personal integrity with the care it deserves as your most precious resource. Sometimes conflicting values come into play when you are trying to protect your sense of personal integrity in your professional role, just as you surely face them in your other roles. For instance, the religious values that led to Janice's position about abortion may come into conflict with values that have led her to become a professional or to take this job in the first place. Her values and beliefs may also mitigate her use of violence and confrontation as forms of resistance.

At the heart of being able to maintain your personal integrity is to know your own values, pay attention to when they are at risk of being compromised, learn to modify them as new insights and experience counsel, and be prepared to defend and weigh them.

THE RESPONSIBILITY TO IMPROVE YOURSELF

Another responsibility is to continue to become a better professional and to learn more about how your professional role provides an opportunity for self-fulfillment and service to others. Each can be viewed as a charge.

The Charge to Remain Competent Professionally

A professional is required to continue to maintain a high level of professional competence by taking continuing education courses and by demonstrating proficiency in other ways. Sometimes relicensure or recertification examinations are required after a number of years to assure that you have kept up your knowledge and skills. Almost all states require you to demonstrate that you have taken steps to engage in lifelong learning professionally. The goal of these requirements is to safeguard your patients, but for most people the idea of being competent on the job is closely related to their feelings of accomplishment and satisfaction too. In that case your self-improvement in professional areas involves consideration of both your patients' and your well-being. Recall Ross's observation that if there were a duty of self-improvement it would flow from the fact that we should bring about as much good overall as we can, including more good for ourselves!

The Charge to Improve Yourself Personally

Beyond improvement in professional areas, there is a charge to improve your personal healthfulness, skills, and interests. Do you have hobbies or other interests? A well-rounded person always makes a better professional insofar as he or she has relief from the demanding routine of professional work. One of the best safeguards against becoming bored or burned out is to have outside compelling interests that require concentrated attention and provide delight. It is not an accident that many application forms for programs of study or jobs include a question about your interests, hobbies, and personal skills unrelated to work.

What are your most cherished ways of spending your time outside of your work and study? Put them in order of priority.

1. _____

2. _____

3. _____

If you could add one thing to this list, what would it be? _____

_____

Put down the year (or, if you foresee getting to it sooner, a month) you plan to be able to engage in these activities more often than you do now.

_____

Describe some things you will have to do between now and then to be able to meet the above goal:

_____

_____

_____

I have heard it said that as part of the professional responsibility of self-improvement you and I have a responsibility to be exemplars in maintaining a healthy lifestyle. An exemplar is someone who demonstrates a quality to an unusually high degree, therefore becoming an example to others. In contrast, a dietitian who is obese because of poor dietary habits, a physically unfit physical therapist, a respiratory therapist who smokes cigarettes, a social worker or psychologist who does not attend to personal emotional problems, or a nurse who consistently gets too little sleep would be soundly criticized on the basis of being a health professional who should "know better." The health professional does know better, knowledge-wise, about the deleterious effects of obesity, unfitness, mental stress, driving oneself, and other abuses or neglects of the body and mind. But what do you think? Should health professionals be more responsible than the general public for maintaining a healthy lifestyle? Yes _____ No _____ Why? _____

_____

I am still thinking through my own position, and this is how I feel about it at the moment:

It is difficult to defend the idea that personal excellence in their field is a special responsibility of health professionals. That position begins to sound too much like a duty to oneself. In contrast, it is an aspiration toward which everyone profitably *could* strive for their own sense of healthiness and well-being. Sometimes people who choose a health profession have it as a component of their own personal values system to be fit, trim, and in good physical and mental health. In this regard a health professional may experience a sense of personal responsibility to continue to improve his or her own healthfulness. In short, health-related improvements can be considered an important component of self-improvement but are not a responsibility as such.

Challenges Regarding Personal Integrity: Vigilance Revisited

We return to the story of Janice K. to complete this chapter and to consider one more facet of a professional's responsibility for self-improvement. Does Janice's predicament have anything to do with her responsibility for self-improvement? The answer is yes because every challenge to her personal values system provides an opportunity not only to act in accord with her beliefs but also to respond optimally. In the preceding discussion you were introduced to the idea that vigilance is required for maintaining personal integrity. It should now be easier to understand how such vigilance will help determine Janice's overall degree of self-improvement as a moral being. Vigilance is alertness, watchfulness. If she is alert to the details of past challenges to her personal integrity and uses them wisely as a teacher to help guide her in what she should do in each new situation, she will have taken advantage of a grand opportunity for improving her odds in the direction of her hoped-for results. In other words, if vigilant, she will be better equipped to respond more effectively, efficiently, and caringly with each new situation. Over time her practiced attention to what works best will better prepare her not only for moral leadership in her profession but also for all of life's difficult choices.

SUMMARY

A focus on the well-being of others often is the sole emphasis in health care ethics. Chapters 6 and 7 propose that to survive ethically requires self-awareness, experiences (and reflection on them), a commitment to living according to your personal values system, vigilance in maintaining personal integrity, and strategies for fulfilling responsibilities to yourself. In Chapter 8 you will have an opportunity to examine how colleagues and the institutional mechanisms for support and accountability in health care are relevant to your survival ethically.

Questions for Thought and Discussion

1. Melissa Y. is a nurse who works in the neonatal intensive care unit. She became distressed in the last month because she is increasingly convinced that one of her longtime colleagues is "siphoning off" some of the narcotic medications intended for the patients. Her personal integrity dictates that she pursue the issue. If you were Melissa, how would you proceed? With whom? Why?

2. Some of the physicians who participated in the Nazi medical experiments testified that their activities did not run counter to their feelings of personal integrity. When asked how this could be, they stated that they were simply "doing their job." Discuss the limits of using an individual's personal conscience, convictions, or understanding of his or her professional role as the ultimate standard of moral judgment. What, if any, higher standard is there? What types of checks and balances do you want to have in place to minimize wrongdoing in an institution or society?

3. Some days it would be better to just stay in bed. Bob started out the day by oversleeping, thereby missing his first patient appointment. When he went out for lunch with Bill, his colleague at work, his car was rear-ended at a stoplight. Now he is treating a patient who has just been diagnosed as having lung cancer. Bob expresses his sympathy regarding this bad news. The patient retorts, "You shouldn't sympathize. It's people like you who are part of the problem! You preach about health, but you smoke like a chimney. If you can't be a better example than this to poor common folks like us, you should get out of the health care field and leave it to someone who knows how to take care of his own health." Bob, who has been fighting the cigarette habit, suddenly feels guilty. He wonders if his smoking really is that bad of an example for his patients. He wants to respond to the patient but can't think of what to say regarding this indictment. Can you help him make an appropriate response? Why do you think your idea is an appropriate remark? Is the patient right?

References

1. Ross, W.D. 1930. *The Right and the Good*. Oxford: The Clarendon Press, pp. 26–27.
2. Niebuhr, H.R. 1963. *The Responsible Self*. New York: Harper & Row.
3. Inge, W. 1968. *The Dark at the Top of the Stairs*. In *Four Plays*. New York: Grove Press, pp. 223–304.
4. Matthew 7:3.
5. Martin, M.W. 1986. *Self Deception and Morality*. Lawrence: University Press of Kansas, pp. 6–30.
6. *Bouvia v. County of Riverside*, 159780. Tr 1238-1250 Sup. Ct. Riverside County, California, 1983.

8

Support and Challenges as a Member of the Health Care Team

Objectives

The student should be able to:

- Describe some major areas of professional life that present ethical challenges as a member of a health care team.
- List five guidelines that are useful in assessing whether a prospective place of employment has good peer support mechanisms for its employees.
- Discuss several reasonable expectations a health professional can have of professional peers.
- Analyze several options open to a health professional who is confronted with role conflicts related to professional and personal relationships.
- Define peer review and assess its usefulness.
- List several types of impairment that health professionals may experience that in severe instances lead to incompetence.
- Discuss some general guidelines on how to gather relevant information regarding an alleged incident of incompetent or unethical professional conduct.
- Identify the moral elements in ethical problems that arise when health professionals observe team members engaging in unethical or incompetent professional conduct.
- Outline the appropriate steps to be taken in a whistle-blowing situation.
- Develop several alternative strategies for dealing with a colleague who is engaging in incompetent or unethical conduct and describe probable outcomes of taking each line of action.

New Terms and Ideas You Will Encounter in This Chapter

Health care teams   Whistle-blowing/whistle-blowers
Supererogatory—beyond duty   Due process (legal)
Peer review

Topics in This Chapter Introduced in Earlier Chapters

TOPIC	INTRODUCED IN	DISCUSSED IN THIS CHAPTER ON
Taking care of yourself as a responsibility	Chapter 6	Page 122
Hippocratic Oath	Chapter 1	Page 136
Faithfulness or fidelity	Chapter 3	Pages 125, 136
Beneficence	Chapter 3	Page 136
Ethical dilemma	Chapter 4	Page 127
Justice or fairness	Chapter 3	Page 128
Six-step process of ethical decision making	Chapter 5	Pages 134–136
Nonmaleficence	Chapter 3	Page 136
Deontology	Chapter 3	Page 136
Utilitarianism	Chapter 3	Pages 128, 136

Introduction

This chapter of Section Two launches a new focus. Up until now you have been considering your role as an individual student or professional. But there are ethical dimensions to other roles you assume too, one of the most interesting being a member of a health care team. There you are working together with other professionals to provide optimally competent care to patients as well as participating in other team activities.

SUPPORT AMONG TEAM MEMBERS

No one who works in the health care setting day in and day out escapes moments of self-doubt, anger, or utter frustration. As you read in Chapters 6 and 7, a lot is expected of you in regard to taking good care of yourself. Even so, at times the involvement in the human suffering of illness and disease is too intense, the responsibilities too arduous, and the challenges too monumental to accommodate the most stouthearted individual. The wear and tear of taxing schedules, patients whose problems seem overwhelming, a day in which everything that can go wrong does, or the awareness that someone is being shortchanged and that there seems to be nothing you can do about it can discourage even the most competent, optimistic person.

Many institutions today recognize the need for peer support mechanisms. In some institutions there is an effort to hold departmental or interdepartmental meetings so that problems may be addressed in a setting in which team members feel unthreatened and supported.[1] This type of arrangement usually improves the working relationships among team members and provides a refuge where individuals can receive needed support. In any department, such arrangements can help to humanize the environment for workers and patients alike.[2]

Many have found it wise when applying for a position in a new health care setting to find out whether there is a support network among team members. To make an assessment, the following guidelines are useful:

1. Inquire of your future employer whether there are team meetings or other sessions at which problems associated with the everyday stresses of health care delivery are discussed or ask how such problems are managed.
2. Ask some of the people you will be working with what they believe to be the sources of the most intense stresses in that environment.
3. Ask some of the people you will be working with how each, as an individual, deals with the stresses of his or her position and whether the environment as a whole is a supportive or a divisive one.
4. Make a mental note of those who appear to be potential sources of support under stress or if no one appears to be.
5. Perhaps most important, try to ascertain whether it will be possible to help change the sources of stress that are changeable and who will help accept responsibility for fostering such change. In other words, is there an attempt to get at structural and other sources of stress and to decrease or eliminate them?

What *other* questions or concerns would you address?

1. _____

_____

2. _____

_____

A setting in which everyone denies that problems exist, or becomes defensive when discussion about them arises, probably signals that stresses are accepted as a "necessary evil," dealt with alone, without the support of colleagues.

If you are already employed, you can help create a greater support network among coworkers by being attentive to the blahs and blues that col-

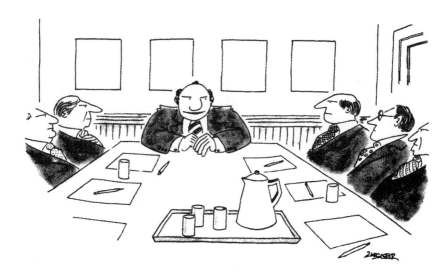

"Of course what we're doing is wrong, but that doesn't make it indefensible."

FIGURE 8–1

leagues seem to be experiencing, to risk sharing your own "dark spaces" with people you judge to be trustworthy, and to make suggestions regarding the need for sessions devoted to working through problems related to the stresses of your working situation. Often knowing that others are experiencing similar frustrations is all that is required to put processes in motion that can turn your loneliness or frustration into an opportunity for learning and growth as a group.

Fortunately it is extremely likely you will be able to find a supportive work setting. Friendships may even take root in the shared experiences, concerns, and time spent with other members of the health care team. A friend you meet in the work situation may become the key figure in building a supportive network, and as friends the two of you can provide support to each other and for others. The joy of discovering and cultivating such a friendship is among the most rewarding of the many fringe benefits of a health professional's career.

Often the ethical dimensions that arise within such friendships or working relationships are similar to those that are inherent in the health professional–patient relationship.[3] For example, telling the truth, honoring confidences, acting with compassion, and respecting the dignity of your colleagues are as important as doing these things for patients. What do you think to be the very minimum support that you should be able to expect from your peers?

_____

_____

_____

I have my own list, based on the ethical element or principle of fidelity or _____ (faithfulness) to each other. As you may recall, faithfulness means that your reasonable expectations will be met. I think it is a reasonable expectation that as a member of the health care team you will provide or encourage and, in turn, will receive:

1. Reassurance regarding questions about good patient care or other professional judgment matters
2. An arrangement in which everyone carries a fair share of the workload
3. Sympathetic understanding of your colleagues regarding work-related stresses
4. An environment conducive to a high level of functioning and one that fosters work satisfaction
5. Mechanisms for the protection of everyone's basic rights
6. Encouragement to everyone to develop both professionally and personally within the work environment
7. Acceptance of responsibility for identifying ways to reduce or eliminate stress-generating situations

As you think of other things you would expect and want to help protect and encourage, be bold in making suggestions to those with whom you work. Sometimes a word well placed can help to increase everyone's imagination about how to work together better as teammates.

With some bases of support having been examined, the remainder of this chapter discusses difficulties that may arise in the course of working as a team member. You will be introduced to three types of challenging situations:

1. The potential for favoritism in settings where it would be inappropriate
2. The opportunity to provide peer review
3. The duty to report unacceptable conduct of a teammate

FRIENDSHIP AND FAVORITISM

Occasionally a close relationship you have with a professional teammate creates a tension you will have to resolve. The story of Maureen Sitler and several of her teammates illustrates one such version of the situation.

THE STORY OF MAUREEN AND DANIELA: FRIENDSHIP V. PROFESSIONAL OBJECTIVITY

Maureen Sitler is the chief respiratory therapist and Director of the respiratory intensive care unit (ICU) of a large university hospital. There are two staff therapists in the unit with her.

Maureen has been on vacation during the past two weeks and arrives home late Sunday night. When she reports to work on Monday morning she finds a note on her desk saying that Karen, one of the two staff therapists, has had to leave town to be with her mother, who has suffered a serious heart attack. She says she will be gone at least this week and maybe next.

The other therapist, Tom Morgane, arrives and brings Maureen up to date on the activities. He assures her that, as usual, the patient load soared immediately after she left and that the unit has been buzzing ever since.

They sort through the present patient load and are relieved that no new patients have come in over the weekend. They decide that between them they can just manage for the day. Suddenly Maureen feels weary, as if she had never been on vacation.

She is writing names of the patients on the schedule board in the office when a unit clerk brings a note to her detailing four patients in other parts of the hospital who need therapy. The note is from the hospital's other respiratory therapy department director, the one who serves the general inpatient population. Often the two directors make such requests of each other when their own loads are overwhelming. Maureen's first reaction is to refuse to accept anymore, but she takes the note to her desk.

The first patient is an 81-year-old widow with inhalation burns. She accidentally started a fire that gutted her kitchen when a kitchen towel caught on fire.

The second referral is a three-year-old child with congenital lung and bronchial deformities. Another repair of the bronchial tubes had been performed.

The third is a 31-year-old woman with severe asthma.

Maureen lays out the three referral sheets in front of her without bothering to locate the fourth and studies the schedule again. At *most* they can accept only one more patient today. She decides to call the other chief therapist, Sandra Haynes, to ask her judgment regarding the relative urgency of these patients.

She is dialing, tapping idly with her forefinger on the one referral she has not yet read, when the name Daniela Green leaps off the page at her. She picks up the referral and reads it again. Her heart begins to pound in her throat. She slams down the receiver and runs to the treatment area where Tom is working. "This can't be *our* Danie," she exclaims in a husky voice. Tom puts a hand on her shoulder, as if bracing himself as well as offering comfort to her. "Didn't you know, Maureen? I wondered why you didn't say anything, but I figured maybe you were too upset to talk about it. She is hospitalized with severe pneumonia."

Maureen feels sick to her stomach. Daniela Green is the chief medical records administrator. Daniela and Maureen often have worked together on committees, and Daniela recently gave an excellent in-service workshop for the physical and respiratory therapy departments. On a number of occasions Maureen and Daniela have attended plays and other social events together. Two years ago they initiated a drive to find some support for improving or, as they put it, "humanizing" the environment of the waiting areas throughout the hospital. Of all her professional colleagues, Maureen feels she can trust Daniela most. On several occasions Maureen has called on Daniela as a "sympathetic ear" and has found her insightful and understanding. During her vacation Maureen had been thinking that she should take the time to cultivate the budding friendship, knowing that it could take root and deepen.

Maureen's first reaction is to squeeze Daniela into the treatment schedule, no matter what. But something stops her. How can she be fair to all involved and still respond to the additional loyalties of friendship she feels toward Daniela?

You will have an opportunity to reflect on this case throughout the chapter because it highlights several types of ethical challenges that you could face—and probably will face—as a team member. The first thing I want to call to your attention is the importance of providing support to and accepting support from each other.

The story of Maureen Sitler illustrates well how easy (and how wonderful) it is to develop friendships in the work place. It is not surprising, considering that we spend some of the best (and if not best, at least the most) hours of our lives at work! Friendships, love relationships, and business partnerships with people you meet first as a team member are all within the realm of possibility. For all of the beauty of such eventualities, undoubtedly some challenges arise because of dual roles you now have with that person.[4]

We will explore the challenges by returning to Maureen's problem. It appears she has an ethical dilemma. To review, briefly describe an ethical dilemma here:

A dilemma is _____

_____

What are two conflicting courses of action Maureen faces as an agent in this situation?

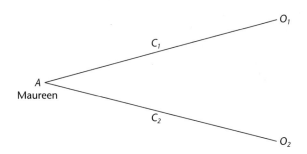

If two do not seem readily apparent, you will have an opportunity to come back to them after you have considered several options Maureen can take in deciding who should be the recipient of her professional services on this day when all of the respiratory therapists are so busy.

There are several options open to her, among them:

1. Accept Daniela Green for treatment because they are friends.
2. Accept Daniela because she is well loved by many people in the hospital and not to give her priority will adversely affect many people at the hospital.
3. *Not* accept Daniela because showing favoritism in such instances is wrong, and it is impossible not to show partiality to someone Maureen knows and respects, likes, or loves.
4. *Not* accept Daniela because she is in less immediate need of this particular health professional's services than the other three patients seem to be.
5. Choose randomly who among the four will be treated today (draw straws).
6. Or, accept the three and treat Daniela after hours.

Can you add others?

7. _____

8. _____

First, let us consider option 1. All things being equal, you would expect a friend or colleague to act favorably on your behalf and would be prepared to do likewise. One evidence of friendship and colleagueship is this type of commitment. If you put yourself in Maureen's shoes, however, it is easy to see that Maureen also experiences a pull to the ideal of treating all patients with equal regard or dignity (the principle of justice). Thus her loyalties are divided. Accepting Daniela for the reason stated in option 1 oversimplifies the ethical problem Maureen is facing because it ignores the reality of conflicting commitments.

Option 2 entails a type of utilitarian reasoning. If Daniela is not accepted for treatment, the morale of the whole hospital will be affected. They will think, "The same thing could happen to me. Would my colleagues overlook me for someone else too?" Maureen might say, along this line of reasoning, "Particular loyalties and justice aside, it just doesn't pay in the long run to accept for treatment those who do not command the sympathies of the hospital the way that Daniela does."

Practically speaking, this type of reasoning often underlies decisions. The VIP treatment goes to the famous, the familiar, and the fearsome. But the moral point of view requires that the various duties experienced in the friendship or health professional–patient relationships not be ignored so facilely. Accepting Daniela for the reason stated in option 2 again oversimplifies the ethical dilemma Maureen is facing.

Option 3 again emphasizes the difficulty of trying to proceed fairly or impartially when you are faced with a decision that involves someone you know and care about. Refusing Daniela treatment primarily because she and Maureen are teammates intuitively seems as unfair as automatically providing privileges because of it. And so, acting on option 3 is not a morally adequate decision either. In contrast, Maureen's idea of telephoning her respiratory therapist colleague, who may know the other patients, is a good plan: The other therapist might provide insight and more balanced judgments regarding unfair biases she would introduce by having a vested interest in her friend's welfare.

The ethical priority in regard to Maureen's dilemma is the health professional–patient relationship rather than her relationship with another team member.[5] Daniela is in this situation because of her medical condition, and her need for Maureen in this instance specifically is the need that a patient experiences in relation to a health professional. Therefore, whether the bonds of friendship are generally more binding than the health professional–patient relationship may be an extremely interesting question, but the governing framework for *this* situation should be the health professional–patient relationship.

Option 4 comes much closer to a decision that takes three important ethical considerations into account

1. The health professional–patient relationship as the proper relationship governing the decision
2. The principle of justice
3. An indication that degree of medical need is the common element by which all three patients can be compared.

More detailed discussion regarding the criteria on which to base distributive justice decisions in health care will be postponed until Chapter 14. Here it is sufficient to point out that the criterion of medical need and Maureen's potential to be of benefit in each case is a reliable guide for the type of decision Maureen must make.[6] Because the patients' needs differ, Maureen does not have to resort to other criteria of selection (option 5).

If Maureen accepts this type of reasoning regarding the proper moral criteria for determining who should be accepted for treatment, it should in no way diminish her desire to expend her best energies for her fellow team member.

Option 6 enables her to do just that. By accepting the others on the basis of their greater medical need she meets the requirements of fairness to the other patients, who get treated instead, but does not prevent Maureen from taking an extra step to help her colleague. Philosophers call Maureen's conduct *supererogatory*, a type of morally praiseworthy conduct that goes beyond duty.[7]

If you listed additional options, take a few minutes and analyze each, using a process similar to the one I used to analyze the other six.

_____

_____

_____

_____

_____

This is one example of a challenging situation that a team member was able to work out. You can see here, as in other areas of professional practice, that the six-step process of ethical decision making provides a framework for systematically thinking through and acting on difficult ethical situations. I have emphasized step 4, the step that requires you to name and think about the practical alternatives or options open to you. But in the process of analyzing the options, I have had to draw on the other steps too:

- Gather relevant information about the story
- Identify the type of problem
- Choose the ethical approach I would use

Having completed steps 1 to 4 I am ready to act and finally to reflect on my action.

In summary, the tension that may develop because of a desire to give preferential treatment to a friend can be successfully weighed against the requirement that you be objective regarding the demands of your role as a professional.

PEER EVALUATION

A second type of ethical challenge to team members arises around the concept of peer evaluation, or *peer review*. Increasingly members of professional organizations, educational institutions, and treatment facilities are being asked to evaluate the quality of their colleague's work and moral character.[8]

Peer review is designed primarily to ensure that the high standards of professional practice agreed on by a group are upheld. The standards may be set by the professional body itself or may be imposed by governmental or other agencies. An identical form is used for evaluation of all individuals similarly situated, and a well-designed form will reflect the extent to which an individual is upholding agreed-on professional standards and goals.

Peer review often generates data that then become a basis for comparisons among similarly situated colleagues. It may be a source that is referred to when salary increases, honors, promotions, or other work-related distinctions are being determined. It also can become a source of evidence when a person is fired, demoted, denied tenure or licensure, or in other ways has negative sanctions imposed.

And so, while the main emphasis in peer review is on its value as a procedure to ensure high-quality functioning in the health professions, it also functions secondarily as a personal profile of a person's progress (or lack of it) in attaining professional stature. With this understanding of peer review, let us consider the story of Maureen Sitler again. But let us add more intrigue to her situation:

THE STORY OF MAUREEN AND TOM: PEER REVIEW CHALLENGE

Maureen and Tom Morgane have not told anyone that they are in love and are planning to be married in the autumn. They are both in their early thirties and wish to remain at the hospital because of the favorable opportunities for advancement and also because they enjoy the part of the country in which they live.

Although both are about the same age, Maureen has worked longer as a respiratory therapist, and everyone agrees that she is exceptionally well qualified as director of the respiratory therapy unit in the ICU. She has written several papers, engaged in clinical studies, and learned some difficult diagnostic techniques through special training.

News has just come out that Sandra Haynes has decided to take a position elsewhere. The hospital administration has decided to unite Maureen's and Sandra's departments into one large hospital department, and a nationwide search will be conducted to find the best person to head this department. Within the hospital itself two people are obvious contenders; Maureen is one. The other is a woman who has been in the other department about as long as Maureen has been in the ICU and who seems equally well qualified.

After the first extensive search is made, four people are still in the running. Both Maureen and the other woman are among them. As part of the administration's attempt to make a wise choice, they now ask several people to submit evaluations of Maureen and the other woman. Tom is among those asked to make this peer evaluation.

Maureen and Tom are elated at the possibility that Maureen may be appointed director of the department. Tom believes not only that she is well qualified but also that she very much wants the position. They both are aware that her substantial increase in salary would be helpful in getting them started and may enable them to put a down payment on a house.

What should Tom do in this situation?

1. He should fill out the form and say nothing about their personal involvement because he believes she is well qualified for the position.
2. He should fill out the form and say nothing about their personal involvement because their personal lives have nothing to do with their professional lives.

3. He should fill out the form, making a note that while he believes she is well qualified, the people reading the form should know that he also is engaged to be married to this woman.
4. He should refuse to fill out the form because it is impossible to make an objective evaluation regarding Maureen's qualifications.

Select your choice here before proceeding.

1. _____   2. _____   3. _____   4. _____

Here is the way I reason about this situation. See if you agree and why:

Tom may think that whatever he says is not going to make a difference anyway. But that is an avoidance of assuming the responsibility he has been asked to assume. From a moral standpoint, he should try to work out a method of acting responsibly while still providing the information needed for the evaluators to assess the possible pitfalls of his attempt to give an objective peer review.

Options 3 and 4 come closest to bringing into focus the awareness that his personal relationship with Maureen makes it more difficult, although not necessarily impossible, to proceed in a manner that acknowledges the conflicting loyalties operating in the situation. As the primary purpose of peer evaluations should be to help maintain the high standards of professional practice, he must do some soul-searching to assure himself that the high esteem he has for Maureen professionally really is based on the high quality of her work and her skills. If he can give a positive response to that issue, he should choose option 3. If there is any doubt, he should choose option 4. He should also discuss his decision with Maureen before doing either. If he chooses option 3, he should document his statement with examples and try especially hard to recall instances in which he was less than enthralled with her professional judgment or skills. Disclosing that he has a vested interest as a friend or fiancé will allow the person reading the review to take into consideration the bias that may be introduced. It is to be hoped that the person reading the review will know that it is difficult enough to evaluate one's peers and that additional difficulty is introduced by their personal relationship.

Even when the added component of friendship or a love relationship is not introduced, peer review by team members can be an emotionally taxing situation. Essentially you are being asked to engage in a process of affirming or discrediting your fellow team members in relation to their professional quality and skills. In the first place, all health professionals have some doubt about their own judgments from time to time, simply because the nature of professional practice is fraught with ambiguities. As a result it is not surprising if you are hesitant to pass negative judgment on someone else's activities, knowing well that everyone has an Achilles heel. Second, there is the fear that if you are too rough on colleagues, the tables may one day be turned. Finally, sometimes there is a loyalty to one's profession that acts as a deterrent to saying anything negative about a member of the profession. Whatever the source of the difficulty, the health professional who assumes this responsibility with a thoughtful, fair, and compassionate approach can help to uphold the high standards of professional practice. In the end it will benefit the peer, the person's patients, and the professions themselves.[9]

As these challenges face many people who agree to conduct peer evaluations, the practice of involving several people in any review helps to mitigate biases and other difficulties. The person who reads all of them (i.e., the administrator, search committee chairperson, or other person) will look for areas of congruence among the several reviewers. If one evaluation is radically out of line with the others, further evaluation may be merited.

BLOWING THE WHISTLE ON UNETHICAL OR INCOMPETENT COLLEAGUES

A challenge of another type arises when there is evidence that a team member is engaging in unethical or incompetent behavior. When such a person is reported, the person or persons making the report are called *whistle-blowers* and their action is called *whistle-blowing*. Consider the following true story, which made national headlines when it happened:

THE STORY OF THE MARCUS BROTHERS

The Marcus brothers were gynecologists practicing at a large teaching hospital in New York City. They had written a leading textbook on gynecology and were highly respected by their colleagues. Numerous women who had been their patients for years expressed great confidence in them as physicians.

In later years, however, both had become addicted to barbiturates. At first the addiction made no perceptible difference in their practice, but eventually it became obvious to colleagues and patients alike that something was wrong. They began to miss appointments and to see patients while they were obviously under the influence of the drugs. Misdiagnosis and poor judgment in treatment were reported repeatedly by patients, but the brothers' colleagues tried to pretend that nothing was wrong. The few who confided their concern to each other did so in vague terms and tried to reassure each other that the men were just going through a difficult time and that soon everything would be back to normal. How long this ostrichlike, head-in-the-sand response continued is not really known. Complaints had been coming in from patients for at least several months. The physicians did not kill any of their patients, which undoubtedly would have brought the problem to a quick focus. But finally their colleagues and the hospital where they worked reported on them, confronting them with their problem and their resulting incompetence to practice. In reporting, the colleagues had engaged in an act that has come to be known as whistle-blowing.

When learning about this case many people, including health professionals, were aghast. How could such negligence and denial go on for so long? As you reflect on this situation, list two or three reasons why you think the physicians' colleagues and the administration failed to act quickly and decisively.

1. _____

2. _____

3. _____

The story of the Marcus brothers and other stories of misconduct, like many ethical problems, can be examined systematically by applying the six-step process described in Chapter 5.

Today, professional organizations, as well as government licensing and disciplinary boards, are acknowledging that instances less (or more) serious than this do occur among all types of health professionals. Offenses include severe substance abuse, the apparent inability to exercise sound professional judgment, severe depression, paranoia or other mental disorders, sexual abuse of patients, theft from patients or institutions, chronic lying, fee splitting, and practicing without a license or under other false pretenses. You need not watch soap operas to know that health professionals include all types of people.

Step 1: Gather Relevant Information

Usually the knowledge of an actual offense committed against patients or colleagues gradually comes to the attention of colleagues. A rumor is heard that Miss Werthheimer, a nursing unit clerk, accused Patient A of threatening to kill her by poisoning her food, and she claims to have reported him to the CIA. Mr. Grabowski, a surgical technician, is said to have reported to work after an unexplained absence of three days with the smell of whisky on his breath and contaminated the surgical suite by not scrubbing in properly. Money has been reported missing from patients' homes after Mrs. Waltham has made a home visit to them. The mother of a young boy accuses Alan DeJong of sexually abusing him during a recent treatment. An old woman claims that Dr. Sakabuto tried to suffocate her with a pillow during the night. Word is out that Mr. Fried forged his papers and is not a graduate of an approved school.

These dramatic cases are the type that hit the newspapers if the wrongdoing is made public. At the same time more common problems arise that are not as dramatic but that potentially are just as dangerous to patients. For instance, take the case of a health professional who has family problems and copes by excessive drinking or abuse of over-the-counter or prescription medications.

These rumors are about people one works with, side by side, consults with, and has eaten lunch or had coffee with for months or years. Even the person who seems rather strange or is considered a loner is more easily dismissed as a curiosity than viewed as an enemy among the ranks. Unfortunately such rumors are more easily believed as carrying a kernel of truth when the person is disliked or suspected in the first place. But, even so, in almost all cases this type of rumor is first met with disbelief by most people. Indeed, to base one's judgment solely on such a report would be morally indefensible behavior.

What should be the response to this type of hearsay information? As in most such situations the information should not be totally denied or ignored, but no judgment against the person should be made on this tenuous ground. The process of gathering relevant information must be taken seriously. The characteristics of the person who makes the complaint should be taken into consideration, but he or she should never be dismissed as senile, crazy, irrational, or otherwise unable to report accurately what has happened. At the very least the person making the complaint should be asked directly for details. A further step is to ask whether he or she is willing to put the complaint into writing. Although this in itself does not render the alleged offender guilty, it is a sign that the person observing the conduct is willing to describe his or her perceptions of the situation in writing and probably would be willing to defend it before a grievance committee or in a court of law if necessary. Hesitance to report someone in cases of a real offense often comes from fear of reprisal from the alleged offender or fear of stigma (e.g., in cases of rape).

In all but the most serious cases it is wise to hold judgment in abeyance as long as the report remains at the level of one report by one person, especially if the person is not willing to put the incident into writing. Almost all institutions now have appropriate processes for reporting suspicious or outright improper conduct. These processes are designed to protect the rights of everyone involved, to provide *due process* under the law, and should be followed rigorously. Of course, neither 2 nor 200 complaints *in themselves* render an alleged offender guilty. For example, in Nazi Germany, health professionals refusing to engage in inhumane medical research on prisoners were condemned as criminals by many other members of the German medical community (except, of course, the members of that community already in prison camps). One would hardly count them guilty!

Step 2: Identify the Type of Ethical Problem

What duties to the patient are the most important in this type of situation?

You might have answered nonmaleficence or beneficence or faithfulness. Any of these is correct. For example, health professionals have a duty to patients to try to ensure that no harm is done to them and to be faithful to their best interests within the health care setting. The colleagues who closed their eyes to the obvious technical incompetencies that the Marcus brothers exhibited because of their addiction clearly breached both of these duties to patients. At the same time, there is a duty to fellow team members to try to ensure that no harm be done to them either. Without trust among colleagues the complex and emotionally taxing tasks involved in providing high-quality health care could not be performed. The Hippocratic Oath views this bond as so fundamental that the first one third of the Oath is devoted to the topic (see Chapter 1). Today the ethical codes and other ethics guidelines of almost all health professions include similar guidelines that address the importance of loyalty among members of the team. Take a minute to peruse the code of ethics of your profession to see what it states.

You can probably quickly identify the type of ethical problem facing health professionals when there are two correct courses of action but to act on one necessarily will compromise the other.

This type of problem is an ethical _____. (If you did *not* answer dilemma, go back to Chapter 4 for a review.)

But in situations of conflict, to whom is one's loyalty more binding, the patient or the colleague? There is broad agreement among those reflecting on such topics that in cases of conflict the health professional's first loyalty must be to patients. Elsewhere I have shown that sometimes the idea of being a member of a health care team might make it difficult to expose a weak or erring member of the team or to give away team secrets.[10] Perhaps admitting that a colleague is in big trouble simply hits too close to home, even though the other members of the team all are aware of the responsibility to do so.

Step 3: Use Ethics Theory or Approaches to Analyze the Problem

Before exploring the alternative courses of action, consider the ethical approach to use. The approach I chose focused on a dilemma in which at least two principles have to be weighed against each other. Therefore I have employed a _____ approach. (If you answered deontological, you have learned well and remember one of the main points in Chapter 3.)

If a utilitarian approach had been employed, you would have weighed the _____ only. Suppose you decided to employ a utilitarian approach. What are some of the potential consequences you would want to take into account in addition to the one stating that the patient would be harmed?

_____

_____

_____

If this discussion of deontology, utilitarianism, duties, and ends seems quite vague, go back and review Chapter 3.

Step 4: Explore the Practical Alternatives

The moral decision to blow the whistle on a fellow team member can be among the most agonizing in your role as a health professional.[11] Psychologically speaking there is tremendous potential for your own ego, beliefs, and hopes to take a battering. The loss of an errant colleague can also signal the loss of a friend or the loss of your belief in an ideal you thought was a shared ideal. Understandably it is a comfort to believe that you will not be faced with such a dilemma, especially if the offender is a close friend. But to hope for such good fortune does not excuse you from trying to prepare for it. Your moral character is always tested. It takes a full dose of wisdom, patience, fortitude, a striving toward justice, much compassion, and a capacity for sympathetic involvement to know when and how to proceed on incriminating evidence when a colleague or friend is implicated. Before reading ahead, list the alternative courses of action you could take.

1. _____
2. _____
3. _____

One alternative in some situations is to stave off a problem before a real offense is committed. For instance, we can speculate that the Marcus brothers might not have reached such a deep state of addiction had they been confronted by a trusted colleague many months earlier and this colleague had confided his or her concern about their behavior changes and offered assistance if needed. An environment of team support emphasized in the earlier discussion of this chapter could have created the tone for early intervention. Often the breaking point between a professional's attempt to maintain self-esteem or professional responsibilities and total resignation to the destructive forces at work within is the realization that colleagues have turned their backs. Most people know when they are in trouble. At the point of greatest need and alienation a direct contact coming from someone who cares enough to confront the problem tactfully can often provide courage for one to seek help and can be the thin thread back to more sound functioning. Whenever possible you ought to act to affirm such a person as someone in a struggle and offer your support. This may include suggesting that the person *not* continue to practice, at least until he or she is on more solid footing. The motivation for risking yourself enough to reach out to a fellow team member in distress often arises from a sense that it could be you in a similar situation and that, in some fundamental regard, we all are in the game together. Many years ago John Donne caught sight of that possibility:

> No man is an Island, entire of itself; every man is a piece of the continent, a part of the main, if a clod be washed away by the sea, Europe is the less . . . any man's death diminishes me, because I am involved in mankind; and therefore never send to know for whom the bell tolls; it tolls for thee.[12]

A second possible course is to do nothing. The shortcoming of this position is that once you have identified the potential problem, doing nothing is also a course of action. When harm to patients is likely to ensue, your neglect has become complicity.

A third course is to act decisively to remove the person from a position in which he or she can do further harm. This is the appropriate course of action once the relevant information has been gathered and analyzed and is persuasive. A secure rule of thumb is to keep the information as contained as possible, use the usual channels of communication as much as possible, and persevere. It is extremely important to honor the alleged violator's privacy, respect, and legal rights, no matter how grievous a "crime" you may think the person has committed.

Unquestionably there are some difficult judgment calls involved in actually taking the final step of whistle-blowing. For instance, if possible you should warn the person that you have reached the point where you plan to call attention to an alleged violation of ethical or legal standards. Also, you should decide whether to talk to anyone else before you act, knowing that sometimes there is safety in numbers and also that your own perceptions may be skewed. Finally, you should give careful attention to whether you have exhausted the other possibilities that may allow you to take a less radical step and still be responsible in your role as a moral agent.

Steps 5 and 6: Complete the Action and Evaluate It

Should you be faced with a whistle-blowing situation, your ability to strike a balance between your sensitivity to the situation and commitment to proceed will be one of the greatest challenges you face as a health professional. The attention you have given to it here will serve you well.

Earlier in this chapter I suggested that an incentive to try to intervene early to prevent this situation is partially from the hope that a colleague would help to rescue you if you were in a similar situation. Once the facts are submitted regarding the alleged violation of ethical or competent conduct, the courage to proceed may come from hoping that a health professional would help save you as a patient from being treated by such a person. Part of good strategy is to determine early where your support system is. Only in the rarest instances will such a support network be missing. Indeed most health professionals when faced with difficult decisions regarding their patients' welfare genuinely are concerned that they choose the best course of action for their patients. A thoughtful and wise approach to your colleagues most often generates a position in which there is shared discussion, strategy, and action.

It is in the heat of challenging situations that certain character traits disposing you to be thoughtful also will help you to know whether and how to proceed. An acute sensitivity to the various people affected, combined with the courage to act and the desire to act compassionately, are useful tools at such a moment.

As always, anytime you take a step as profound as whistle-blowing, every step should be reflected on and evaluated after the fact.

SUMMARY

This chapter focuses on several sources of support professionals have and can offer as members of a health care team. The challenge of remaining ethical in peer evaluation situations was discussed as well as serious challenges that arise when a colleague is engaging in unethical or illegal behavior. In the latter situation the person may be ill, extremely stressed, addicted, or devious. Whatever the cause, your motive for considered action is to protect patients, clients, or even society from the harm such a person may cause. If your institution has developed guidelines about unethical or incompetent conduct, use them as aids. If not, you can contribute greatly to the constructive functioning of the institution by helping to develop policies and procedures that will enable potential whistle-blowers to (1) document carefully, (2) maintain due process judiciously, (3) provide as much support all around as possible, and (4) persevere to the completion of the review. Completion probably will involve the role of several others, such as administrators, regulatory board members, risk managers, or designated people in professional associations. The actual personnel and processes will vary. Your job in seeing the issue to completion is to work diligently within prescribed institutional mechanisms.

Questions for Thought and Discussion

1. Uri is one of your colleagues. You and Uri enjoy a good working relationship, although you do not know much about his personal life outside of the work situation. You notice that during the past few days he has become increasingly irritable toward you. You wonder if it is something you have said or done that is making him angry.

   a. What steps, if any, should you take to address this issue?

   _____

   _____

b. Would it make any difference in how you proceed if it appears that his attitude is interfering with the quality of his work? Yes _____ No _____ Why?

_____

_____

c. What criteria would be useful for judging how far to pursue the issue?

_____

_____

2. You are asked to give a job recommendation for your friend Arthur. You have worked with Arthur for over a year on the same health care team and feel qualified to provide such a recommendation. Arthur is an energetic, fun-loving person, and you enjoy his friendship. His manner with patients is sometimes disturbing to you, however. He seems careless at times, almost to the point of incompetence. Quite honestly you would have to recommend him with qualification for the position for which he is applying.

   a. Why would you agree or refuse to provide a recommendation?

   _____

   _____

   b. Do you have a responsibility to your friend to tell him that you are giving him a "qualified" recommendation? Yes _____ No _____ Why or why not?

   _____

   _____

   c. Do you have a responsibility to tell the party requesting the recommendation that you and Arthur are friends? Explain your position.

   _____

   _____

3. Dr. Heisler is a physician in the hospital where Ms McKenzie, a nurse, works. He is admitted to the hospital as a patient about 7 PM complaining of chest pain and is seen by a colleague, Dr. Phillips. Several hours later Dr. Heisler calls Ms McKenzie, the head nurse on the unit, into his room and asks her for a sleeping pill. She says that Dr. Phillips did not order a sleeping pill, ostensibly because Dr. Heisler said he did not need one. Dr. Heisler says that now he needs one. Should she give it to him from the large supply of sleeping pills in her supply room? Defend why or

why not, drawing on the duties, rights, and role issues discussed in your reading so far.

---

4. It was stated in this chapter that option 2 (accepting Daniela because the other hospital personnel would expect it) fails to consider fully all the duties incumbent on Maureen. Surely there are some instances, however, in which *not* showing favoritism to a particular individual may have such dire consequences that favoritism is the alternative that will bring about the best consequences overall. Give some examples.

1. _____

2. _____

3. _____

5. Describe some areas of difference and similarity between the health professional–patient relationship and the relationship that exists between two friends.

---

6. Barbara S. and Joan B. are two health professionals who work together in a large hospital. Both are in their late twenties and have worked together for the last three years. Although they enjoy a friendship at work, their personal lives are so different they do not often socialize outside the hospital.

During the month of March, Barbara notices an aloofness in Joan. They used to share coffee breaks and lunch, but Joan now makes excuses. Joan now seems too busy to talk to Barbara. Barbara is upset and approaches Joan regarding the matter. During the conversation, Joan begins to cry. She confides to Barbara that her husband has been fired from his job. Joan is embarrassed and worried. The pile of bills is growing fast, and the tension in her married life is mounting. Joan is terrified that the others will find out and asks Barbara not to tell anyone. Barbara reassures her: She tells Joan that her secret is safe and offers to help in any way she can.

During the first two weeks in April things get worse. Joan calls in sick several times, and Barbara covers. Several times Joan is late and on two occasions leaves immediately after lunch. Joan's work is being left undone, and others are bearing the brunt of her errors. Barbara feels taken advantage of. She has done Joan's work and even lied to the director regarding Joan's whereabouts.

One day over lunch two of the others in their unit start complaining about Joan. They say they are tired of her getting away with things. One has recently had to cover Joan's work on a sick day and says that things were a mess. They tell Barbara that they are going that afternoon to talk to the director. Barbara is upset. What should she do?

---

7. You are told by a patient whose complications from delivery required her to remain hospitalized on the OB ward that Dr. Redmarck is acting "inappropriately" toward her. She says she is scared, and she looks it. When you ask what she means, she says, "Twice this week he has stopped in during the late evening and has asked to examine my breasts. At first I didn't think anything about it, but then I started thinking that it didn't have anything to do with my condition. . . . He pulls the covers way back, and lifts up my gown. There's something strange. I dread seeing him." What steps would you take in response to this information?

---

8. You have been asked by the institution where you work to be on a policy committee dealing with whistle-blowing. Outline the steps that you think should be included in a policy document designed to protect all parties involved in a whistle-blowing situation.

References

1. Curtis, K.A. 1994. Attributional analysis of interprofessional role conflict. *Social Science and Medicine* 39(2):255–263.
2. Brahams, D. 1998. Bad professional relations and risks to patients. *The Lancet* Aug 27, pp. 519–520.
3. Purtilo, R. 1995. Professional patient relationship: Ethical aspects. In Reich, W. (Ed.). *Encyclopedia of Bioethics* (2nd ed., vol. 4). New York: Macmillan, pp. 2094–2103.
4. Kagel, J.D., Giebehausen, K.B. 1994. Dual relationships and professional boundaries. *Social Work* 39(2):255–263.

5. Veatch, R.N., Flack, H.E. 1997. *Case Studies in Allied Health Ethics*. Upper Saddle River, NJ: Prentice-Hall, pp. 53–54.
6. Pellegrino, E., Thomasma, D. 1988. *For the Patient's Good: The Restoration of Beneficence in Care*. New York: Oxford University Press.
7. Feinberg, J. 1961. Supererogation and rules. *Ethics* 71:39–46.
8. Purtilo, R. 1995. Teams-health care. In Reich, W. (Ed.). *Encyclopedia of Bioethics* (2nd ed., vol. 3). New York: Macmillan, pp. 2469–2472.
9. Fagin, C.M. 1992. Collaboration between nurses and physicians: No longer a choice. *Academic Medicine* 67(5):285–303.
10. Purtilo, R. 1994. Interdisciplinary health care teams and health care reform. *Journal of Law Medicine and Ethics* 22(2):121–126.
11. Cannon, B.L., Brown, S.S. 1988. Nurses' attitudes towards impaired colleagues. *Image: Journal of Nursing Scholarship* 20(2):96–101.
12. Donne, J. 1623. *Devotions XVII*.

Ethical Dimensions of the Professional-Patient Relationship

9

Confidentiality

Objectives

The student should be able to:
- Define "confidential information" and "confidentiality."
- Identify the relationship of a patient's legal right to privacy with his reasonable expectations regarding confidential information.
- Discuss the values involved in keeping professional confidences.
- Describe how the telling and keeping of secrets is relevant to the understanding of the importance of confidentiality.
- Identify four premises on which the justification for confidentiality rests.
- Discuss the ethical norms involved in keeping and breaking professional confidences.
- Name five general legal exceptions to the professional standard of practice that confidences should not be broken.
- Consider practical options that a professional can take when faced with the possibility of breaking a confidence.
- Discuss some important aspects of documentation that affect confidentiality.

New Terms and Ideas You Will Encounter in This Chapter

Confidential information	Secrets
Confidentiality	Trust
Right to privacy	Computerized medical records

Topics In This Chapter Introduced in Earlier Chapters

TOPIC	INTRODUCED IN	DISCUSSED IN THIS CHAPTER ON
Hippocratic Oath	Chapter 1	Page 148
Beneficence	Chapter 3	Page 152

Introduction

In this and the next several chapters you will have an opportunity to think about specific ways in which patients or clients learn to put their trust in you. You already have met some patients through the case studies that have been presented to help focus your thinking, and in Chapter 7 you considered ways to make the health care environment as welcoming as humanly possible for such people. The idea of confidentiality in health care goes way back. For instance, the Hippocratic Oath, written in the fourth century BC, says,

> And whatsoever I shall see or hear in the course of my profession, as well as outside my profession . . . if it be what should not be published abroad, I will never divulge, holding such things to be holy secrets.[1]

And so confidentiality is a splendid place to begin this focus on your role as care giver to patients or clients.

The based-on-fact story of Maria Garcia, an occupational therapist, and Mark Cohen, a patient, helps set the stage for our discussion.

THE STORY OF MARIA GARCIA AND MARK COHEN

Maria Garcia works as an occupational therapist in the student center of a large university. Her patients are primarily outpatients who are students, faculty, or on the staff of the university.

Mark Cohen, a 29-year-old graduate student in architecture, has been coming to the treatment center three times a week for five weeks. He is receiving exercises for weakness in his right arm and hand, the last remaining symptoms in his upper extremities from a car accident that partially severed his spinal cord. He walks with crutches and long leg braces. Initially he was almost totally paralyzed, but now, several months later, he has recovered almost all function in his arms and trunk.

Ms Garcia knows that Mark Cohen has a history of mental illness, although physically he has been in good health. The nurse practitioner who examined him when he first presented to the health service learned by his own report that he had been hospitalized "in an insane asylum" as a teenager. The nurse practitioner called the registrar's office of the university and learned that his original medical report, filed by his family physician before his admission, reported a history of paranoid schizophrenia that had required hospitalization on four occasions. In each instance he had become delusional, believing that a being from another planet was trying to kill him with a laser beam. There was no record of further problems since he entered the university four years ago or during his under-graduate career at another university. The nurse practitioner recorded this infor-mation on the chart that Maria Garcia received when Mark's treatment began.

When they began working together on his treatment, at first Mark talked animatedly to Maria about such things as his studies, the woman he lives with, and his recent part in a play presented by the local repertory theater group. But with each visit Ms Garcia notes that he becomes less talkative and more with-drawn. He seems to be increasingly depressed.

One Wednesday he arrives late for treatment. He appears preoccupied as he comes through the door and nearly bumps into a woman just leaving the de-partment. When Ms Garcia is about halfway through his treatment, he breaks his sullen silence. "Can you keep a secret?"

Maria, happy to have him communicating again, replies, "Yeah. Sure, I can keep a secret."

"I got her."

"What? I beg your pardon?"

Mark jerks his hand away and says, with great deliberation, "YOU HEARD WHAT I SAID." Then he gazes intently into the palm of his contractured hand and says, "You might not hold a pencil, baby, but you do nice work with a pistol!"

Maria looks around to see if anyone else is witnessing this conversation. No one is. "Mark," she says, her voice controlled, "What are you talking about?"

With this, Mark seems to snap out of his "state" and lets his hand drop back onto the treatment table. His face mellows, and he says, "Oh. I thought I'd play a little joke on you, Maria. Forget what I said—it was only a joke."

Maria studies Mark's face. She decides to push for more information. "Well, I don't like those kinds of jokes. If that's your idea of a joke, I don't find it very entertaining. And if you aren't joking, I think the sooner you turn yourself in, the better off you'll be."

He smiles at her mischievously. She begins to feel angry, and the anger is unmistakable in the tone of her next statement. "Anyone who says 'I got her' and in the next breath talks about a pistol doesn't exactly send me into gales of laughter."

A cloud settles over Mark's face, and she can see that he is withdrawing again. Now, for the first time, she begins to feel frightened. "Mark," she ventures tentatively, "Are you O.K.? Do you need help?"

He replies, "Yeah, I'm O.K. Except maybe for a big exam tomorrow, I'm O.K." Then he adds, teasingly, "You want to take the test for me?"

They complete the session without any further exchange, and he leaves with the promise of being back on Friday. She wishes him well on his exam.

Once he is gone, her first impulse is to telephone the police. But, on second thought, she wonders if it would be better to call the nurse practitioner who took the history, or call her friend Linda who works in medical technology upstairs, or just keep quiet. She hasn't telephoned anyone by the time the next patient arrives and finds her sitting at her desk, deep in thought.

This somewhat extreme-sounding story is based on a real life situation. As is often the case with real life situations in the health care world, there are a number of unanswered questions. In Chapter 5 you learned that knowing how to proceed in the actual situation first involves a fact-finding component. Obviously it is important to know whether Mark has just murdered a woman or shot a rabbit, is teasing Maria, or is delusional. But in order to clarify what has occurred, Maria's ability to obtain further information eventually may require that she break her promise to Mark to "keep a secret" between them.

WHAT IS CONFIDENTIAL INFORMATION AND CONFIDENTIALITY?

Can you define "confidential information"? Try to do so here:

_____

_____

The most commonly accepted idea of *confidential information* in the professions is that it is information about a patient or client that is harmful, shameful, or embarrassing. Does it necessarily have to come directly from that person? No. Information that is furnished by the patient directly, or comes to you in writing or through electronic data, or even from a third party might count as confidential.

Who is to be the judge of whether information is harmful, shameful, or embarrassing? The person himself or herself is the best judge, but any time you think a patient has a reasonable expectation that sensitive information will not be spread around, it is best to err on the side of treating it as confidential. Of course, as Figure 9–1 illustrates, it is possible to go to extremes so that the best interests of the patient are lost in the process.

A good general rule regarding potentially confidential information is to treat caution as a virtue.

Sometimes the notion of confidential information is discussed within the framework of the constitutional *right to privacy*.[2] It is not incorrect to do so because the right to privacy means that there are aspects of a person's being into which no one else should intrude. At the same time, confidential information creates a situation a little different than that.

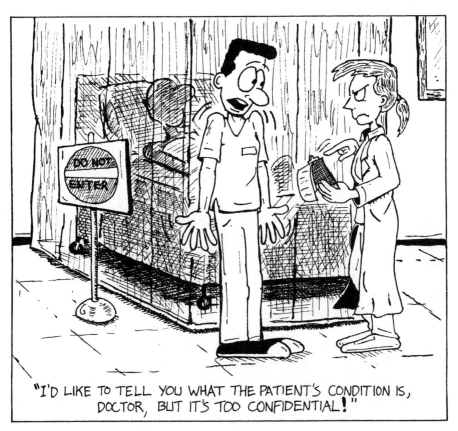

"I'D LIKE TO TELL YOU WHAT THE PATIENT'S CONDITION IS, DOCTOR, BUT IT'S TOO CONFIDENTIAL!"

FIGURE 9–1

The patient who shares private information has chosen to relinquish his or her privacy within bounds; that is, he or she has the reasonable expectation that that information will be shared with certain people to further his or her welfare but that it will be shared with no one else.[3] I may want to tell you something very private, perhaps something I'm ashamed of, because I think you need to know it to plan what is best for me. But I do not want or expect you to spread the word around.

When you have confidential information from patients, they have a right to expect that you will honor your professional promise of confidentiality.

Confidentiality is the practice of keeping harmful, shameful, or embarrassing patient information within proper bounds. Confidentiality always involves a relationship (while privacy does not). It is the most longstanding dictum in health care codes of ethics. Go to the ethics code or other guidelines for your profession and write down here what it says about confidentiality:_____

_____

_____

Developmental theorists tell us that concern about confidentiality begins when a child first is experiencing a desire to keep or tell *secrets*. Secrets manifest a developing sense of self as separate from others, and the desire to share secrets is an expression of reaching out for intimate relationships with others. How secrets are handled in those early stages of development can have longlasting effects on an individual's sense of security, self-esteem, and success at developing intimacy.[4] The *power* of a secret, or of being in a position to tell a secret, is nowhere conveyed more clearly than when a two-year-old has a secret pertaining to someone's birthday present! When was the last time that you had a secret that was so potent it was difficult, maybe impossible, to keep it?

From the standpoint of a health professional's moral obligations and patients' rights, name three principles that will help guide your thinking about your conduct in regard to keeping confidences:

The duty of _____

The duty of _____

The right of _____

If you answered beneficence, nonmaleficence, or fidelity and the right to autonomy, you are grasping the ethical principles or elements supporting confidentiality.

In summary the immediate aims of treating confidential information with utmost care are to:

1. Facilitate the sharing of sensitive information with the goal of helping the patient
2. Exclude unauthorized people from such information

It is not considered a breach of confidentiality if you share this information with other health professionals involved in the patient's care as long as the information has relevance to that case.

_____

KEEPING CONFIDENCES

In Chapters 2 and 3 you were introduced to the ideas of caring and the character traits that a health professional should cultivate. Keeping secret information that flows from patient to health professional is not valued as an end in itself but rather as an instrument that serves *trust*. And the ultimate value that both the keeping of confidences and the subsequent building of trust points to is human dignity.

Keep confidences
   to
Build trust into the relationship
   to
Maintain patients' dignity

Name some character traits or virtues you think would help to serve this end: _____

_____

_____

To decrease trust is to cause harm. Understandably, when there are no conflicts, the health professional will be motivated to keep the confidences entrusted to him or her because it has long been understood that a trusting health professional–patient relationship must be built. Confidentiality serves as one cornerstone for that solid foundation. Bok summarizes four premises on which confidentiality can be justified:

1. Individual autonomy over personal information requires it if we respect individuals' right to have secrets.
2. It presupposes the legitimacy not only of having personal secrets but also of sharing them and assumes respect for intimacy among human beings.
3. The silence creates an obligation beyond the respect due to persons and existing relationships. A promise of secrecy means giving up freedom of action both in giving and in the promise to perform some action. Promises of secrecy are unusual in both respects.
4. There is a utility in professional confidentiality that goes beyond ordinary loyalty.[5]

The fact that conflicts do arise, however, in regard to keeping patient confidences is reflected in a number of codes of ethics. Many codes of ethics today contain statements similar to this one from the American Medical Association (AMA) Principles of Medical Ethics:

A physician shall respect the rights of patients, of colleagues and of other health professionals, and shall safeguard patient confidences within the constraints of the law.[6]

In such statements the conflict is presented as one in which the health professional's duty to refrain from harming a patient (by breaking confidences) is pitted against the duty to prevent harm to someone else, to the patient, or to society. What type of ethical problem does this situation present?

If you answered "an ethical dilemma" and, in the case of breaking a confidence for the patient's own good, "paternalism," you are correct. Try to sketch out the dilemma using the story of Maria and Mark. You take Maria's position.

A = you, the moral agent
C_1 = a course of action leading to patient Mark's well-being
C_2 = another course of action leading to another good end

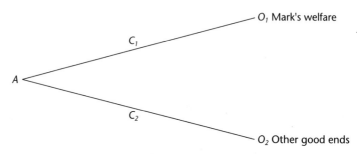

Because these conflicts often arise, the next section addresses the question of when, how, and why confidences may be broken.

BREAKING CONFIDENCES

Most would agree that in certain cases the morally right action involves breaking the patient's confidence. Historically such cases have been exposure of carriers of contagious diseases.

Today, AIDS poses great challenges to confidentiality.

Legal exceptions to the standard of practice that confidences cannot be broken except with patient's consent or at the patient's request include

1. An emergency
2. Patient is incompetent or incapacitated
3. To protect third parties
4. When required by law (e.g., sexually transmitted diseases, child or other abuse)
5. When requesting commitment or hospitalization of a psychiatrically ill patient[7]

In general you must not share confidential information unless it is authorized by the law or by the patient personally. The presumption is that health professionals will try to minimize the number of exceptions. Most patients do not know about the limits of confidentiality. It is a good practice to advise them before rather than after they have divulged sensitive information. From a *legal* point of view, which of these criteria seem to apply to

Maria's predicament? (Obviously more data is needed to make a *conclusive* judgment.)

Returning to the ethical analysis of Maria's story, what *options* does she have in trying to discern what to do?

One way that Maria can handle this situation is to keep the confidence by sharing it with another health professional. Often a health professional's inability to assess whether a person outside the health care setting should be given information leads the professional to discuss it with a trusted colleague first. For Maria, one person seems to be the obvious choice: the nurse practitioner who knows Mark. Maria can also break the confidence by sharing it with a health professional not involved in Mark's treatment, her friend Linda. Part of the motive of this discussion among professionals would be to clarify whether Mark is imminently dangerous to others and ought to be reported to the police.

More often, however, the motive for this type of in-house discussion is to determine whether further medical action on behalf of the patient should be taken. This is the type of situation that the AMA (and many other) codes have in mind when they suggest that breaking the confidence may "become necessary in order to protect the welfare of the individual." In Mark's case, Maria's colleagues may agree wholeheartedly that Mark's comments and behavior are troubling enough that they should not be ignored. They may suggest that Maria recommend Mark make an appointment to see one of the health center psychiatrists. The suggestion could be put in such a way as to assure him that it is her concern for him that prompts the suggestion. It may be exactly what Mark needs. If his comments and behavior continue and he refuses to seek help, however, they may urge Maria to consider a third option: to intervene more directly by helping to arrange for one of the psychiatrists to meet with Mark and Maria during the treatment time. Mark's reactions to these types of interventions will probably clarify much in Maria's mind as to whether Mark indeed was "joking" and, if not, what the problem is.

In sharing her distress with professional colleagues the confidence is kept and possibly eventually broken to benefit the patient himself and not to protect society. Of course, in these types of situations, one of the health professionals may take the initiative of calling the police or may suggest other actions not directed solely to the benefit of the patient. In sharing confidential information in the first place a health professional risks actions being taken by others who are made privy to the information.

Another option for Maria would be to say nothing but to make a note of the conversation on the patient's record. Do you think this is a good idea? Yes _____ No _____

It breaks the confidence of the patient without taking any direct action to foster resolution of a possible problem. Although it may relieve the health professional's anxiety, at least momentarily, it often serves little useful moral purpose in regard to helping the patient. Indeed it is impossible to know who will become privy to the information. Usually this type of action creates more problems than it solves.

Maria does not need to share the information with anyone. She can pretend she was never a party to this conversation and do as Mark instructed, "Forget what I said." But there is yet a fifth option possible. Her decision to keep the conversation between her and Mark in confidence does not commit her to inaction. If she wants to pursue the issue, the one and only person to pursue it with is Mark himself. It may be that the help Mark needs (if any) can be handled just as well, if not better, by further discussion between her and Mark alone. The amount of clarification she can get from other professionals may be minimal, and to obtain their perceptions (based on the "facts," as she has reported them) she must break the confidence she shares with Mark.

It is quite possible that by going directly back to Mark and revealing to him in a supportive way that the conversation was deeply troubling to her, she will gain better insight into the seriousness of his comments. It is probable that if he is suffering from mental stress, he will be willing to seek help. But at least he will know that as he chose to proceed as he did (in asking her to "keep a secret"), Maria did not take his subsequent statement lightly.

Some will insist that the risk is too great. Mark may be a psychotic killer who already has taken another life. Some will prefer that at least one other health professional be told of the situation, as it is potentially violent. This case, like many we discuss, does not admit of simple answers. It would seem, however, that, given the ambiguities involved, for Marcia to begin by immediately breaking the patient's confidence around a single incident such as this compromises the trust that must continue to underlie the relationship between the single health practitioner and patient, especially at a time when this type of relationship is being threatened by changes in the structure of health care. Few would condemn Maria for telephoning another health professional or even the police. But, as the story is told here, it seems that she first can do more to learn from Mark exactly what is going on.

In conclusion, breaking confidences always entails at least one harm, that of creating distrust in the health professional–patient relationship. Two questions I always ask when faced with such a dilemma are:

1. When is the harm of threatening the fragile trust in the relationship outweighed by the benefit?
2. How can the amount of harm be kept to a minimum when it becomes ethically appropriate to break a confidence?

The burden of proof is always on the health professional to minimize the harm.

CONFIDENTIALTY AND MEDICAL RECORDS

Another aspect of confidentiality raised in this story is the process of information sharing and record keeping that goes on within the health care (and other institutional) systems. For example, Mark's diagnosis of paranoid schizophrenia is in his permanent file at the university, in spite of the fact that he has not been hospitalized since he was a teenager for treatment of the condition. There are many unanswered questions about this report, given in the general terms that the family physician reported them. Already the potentially damaging information has been transferred to Mark's medical record by the nurse practitioner. Receiving the information (which we have to assume was quoted accurately from the university file and recorded accurately by her) involved only a phone call. Now a diagnosis of a severe form of mental illness is on two of Mark's permanent records.

The issue of how far this information should and can go takes on greater importance when one considers modern *computerized systems of record keeping*. Virtually all major health care institutions and agencies today use computerized data sheets that enable easy retrieval of almost any information.[8] Depending on what is requested and the policies of the university, the information regarding Mark's history of mental illness may be released to insurance agencies, other universities, federal registries of mental disease, people conducting research, or future employers. In short, Mark is in danger of being *labeled* because of the diagnosis on his record. Maria must be aware that if she records their discussion, Mark's intimations of violence combined with an intimation of mental derangement is a highly stigmatizing profile.

Although ethics as expressed in the codes of ethics of most health professions require that information about patients be kept confidential unless some strongly overriding argument for disclosure exists, the realities of modern health care make this almost impossible. As noted previously, these charts are accessible to many different people and agencies, for many different reasons, and computerized data systems compound the problem. Thus any information that may impair the patient's ability to function freely and confidently in society must be carefully weighed before it is recorded in the medical record.

The medical record is an extremely useful document for health professionals, however. If information about the patient is true and is relevant to his or her health care, then that information ought to be recorded there. If Mark is actually having a recurrent psychotic episode, his previous history of psychiatric hospitalization is highly relevant information. Frequently, however, people who are not qualified to make psychiatric diagnoses do so in their effort to emphasize difficult or aberrant patient behavior.

One example of this is the story of a middle-aged woman with crippling arthritis who was hospitalized at a university hospital where many invasive and dangerous procedures were carried out to evaluate a problem of incipient renal failure. There were many doctors writing the orders for these tests, and none of them bothered to explain to her what was being done or why. She became fearful, then hysterical, claiming that she could trust none of her doctors and that they were trying to kill her. She left the hospital against medical advice, and the intern writing her case summary included "acute paranoiac behavior" as one of the notations. Thus her subsequent encounters with health professionals were strongly influenced by this incorrect and strongly prejudicial statement that was recorded permanently on her medical record. She had no knowledge that it was there and no easy recourse for having it removed.

In this case the patient was harmed by information in the record that was untrue. True information can also be harmful to a patient and, unless it is relevant to the health care of that person, should not be recorded. For example, a 62-year-old man hospitalized after a stroke was lying in bed and overheard two health professionals outside his room discussing how he had suffered his stroke while "getting it on" with his wife. He was embarrassed and angry and refused to accept their treatment attempts after that. It made him distrustful of all the other health professionals involved in his care, as he was sure that such gossip was not limited to the two whose conversation he had overheard. The information was written as part of his admitting history and physical: "The patient suddenly lost the function of his right arm and leg while having intercourse with his wife." This information is *not* relevant to his medical care and should not have been recorded on his chart. His privacy should have been respected in that regard, and the principle of confidentiality extended to excluding it from the medical record. Sexual activity or habits are sometimes relevant to medical care (as, for example, in the case of sexually transmitted disease or sexual dysfunction), but if the information is not relevant, it need not and should not be recorded. In any case, such information should not be fodder for idle gossip in hospital corridors.

As you return to the story of Mark, then, it is important to recognize the great power of the information about your patients or others. Three guidelines are applicable:

1. Untrue information should not be recorded, and questionable information should be clearly labeled as questionable.
2. True information that is not relevant should not be recorded.
3. Information should be handled among health professionals with regard for the privacy and dignity of patients.

Information recorded in the medical record can be of great help or harm to the patient. For this reason the medical record needs to be treated with a great deal of respect. Medical record administrators and others who work in record keeping are usually highly aware of the power of these documents. They function as the gatekeepers for the records and rightfully take great pains to keep the records in order and to make sure that they are available to those professionals who need them and who have a right to see them. Conversely, they also need to be careful that the records are not abused or released to unauthorized persons. Working in the field of medical records can therefore also present difficult ethical dilemmas.

CONFIDENTIALITY AND GENETIC INFORMATION

Genetic information has raised many new ethical issues. None pose greater challenges than those surrounding the traditional guidelines regarding confidential information.[9] The story of Gina's situation raises some questions for you to ponder as you continue to study this book and think about your role as an ethical health professional in the emerging "geneticized" era of health care.

GINA AND THE DISCOVERY OF A BREAST CANCER GENE

Gina Backstrom, a married, 42-year-old Omaha woman, has been in excellent health. Last year she ran the Grandma's marathon in Duluth, Minnesota. She enjoys being an at-home mom with her two teenaged daughters, although she also looks forward to going back to her work as a lawyer when they begin school. Gina comes to her HMO physician now, worried because her sister, Carla, who is four years older than she is, has been diagnosed with carcinoma of the breast.

In their discussion as sisters, Gina and Carla began wondering whether their mother's death of ovarian cancer at the age of 42 was related to her sister Carla's cancer. Gina calls an aunt and verifies that in fact two of their maternal aunts did die of cancer, one of breast cancer and one of ovarian cancer.

Her physician refers her to a physician who is a worldwide expert in breast ovarian cancer syndrome. The counselor at the second physician's genetics unit tells her about *BRCA1* testing and that this could help to clarify for her whether she has the gene. She is further told that if she has the syndrome, there is an 85% to 90% lifetime risk of bilateral carcinoma. She also is advised that if she has the syndrome, she can have a prophylactic oophorectomy because the risk for ovarian carcinoma is 44% to 60% and there are poor screening mechanisms for ovarian cancer. She agrees to go ahead with the tests.

Among the many questions you should be asking are:

1. What are the major ethical issues the physician, the counselor, and Gina face?
2. Now that Gina has chosen to have the tests, should she be required to learn the results? What is her right regarding refusal of results should she change her mind?

3. Should the testing clinic be required to advise her beforehand of pos-sible insurance discrimination and the difficulties that some women have had in accepting this information?
4. If she asks the physician to keep this information from her husband, should the family physician comply since he is the physician for the whole family in their HMO plan?
5. Is she morally obligated to allow the physician to break the news to her 17- and 20-year-old daughters?

The issues of confidentiality are beginning to give rise to practices, law, and policies explicitly designed to provide guidance.[10] In this emerging area of health care you should pay special attention to how you can best protect patient confidentiality while being aware that there may be others whose lives are affected dramatically by the presence of genetic conditions in one member of the family.

SUMMARY

The questions surrounding the practice of keeping patient confidences are not easily resolved. Keeping confidences is a general ethical guideline that the health professional can rely on to maintain trust and foster dignity in the health professional–patient relationship. Sometimes, however, the interests of another person or of society or even the best interests of the pa-tient seem to advise against keeping the confidence.

Current methods of record keeping and information sharing raise addi-tional, difficult questions related to confidentiality. As a health professional you must rely on your considered judgment regarding the various moral obligations of professional practice, the rights of all involved, and the char-acter traits that enable you to maintain a relationship of trust in order to ar-rive at a decision on how to proceed.

Questions for Thought and Discussion

1. The story of Mr. Shaw provides a good basis for thinking about some of the things you have just learned.

Ann von Essen is a health professional, and David Shaw, a patient in the hospital where she works, has been referred to her for discharge plan-ning.

Mr. Shaw, 42 years old, is a pleasant man whose family often is at his side during visiting hours. He was admitted to the hospital with numer-ous fractures and a contusion following an automobile accident in which his car "skidded out of control and hit a tree." He has no memory of the accident, but the person traveling behind him reported the scene.

The arrangement for his discharge is going smoothly. During one of Ann von Essen's visits, however, Mr. Shaw's mother, a wiry old woman of about 80, follows her down the corridor. At the elevator, Mrs. Shaw says, "I wish you'd tell sonny not to drive. It's those fits he has, you know. He's had 'em since he was a kid. Lordy, I'm scared to death he's going to kill himself and someone else too."

Ann is at a loss as to what to say. She thanks Mrs. Shaw and jumps on the elevator. She goes down the elevator for one flight, gets off, and runs back up the stairs to the nurses' desk. She reads Mr. Shaw's chart and finds nothing about any type of seizures.

Put yourself in the place of Ann von Essen. Do you have confidential information? What should you do? Why?

Let us assume that in the state in which you work the law requires that people suffering from epileptic seizures be reported to the department of public health, which in turn reports this to the department of motor vehicles.

a. What do you think is the morally "right" action to take regarding Mr. Shaw once you have become the recipient of this information?

b. What duties and rights inform your decision about what to do?

2. Suppose you believe that it is morally right for the department of motor vehicles to be advised of this situation. The obvious course of action is for you to inform the physician, the physician to report to the public health department, and for them to report to the department of motor vehicles. If any of the usual links in this process are broken by failure to communicate the information, do you have a responsibility to make sure the department of motor vehicles has actually received this information? Defend your position regarding how far you believe you and anyone else in *your* profession should go in pursuing this matter.

References

1. Hippocrates. The Oath. In *Hippocrates I* (translated by W.H.S. Jones, The Loeb Classic Library). 1923. Cambridge, MA: Harvard University Press, pp. 299–301 (quote p. 301).

2. *Griswold v Connecticut*. 1965. 381 U.S. 479. 85 S Ct. 1678.
3. Smith-Bell, M., Winslade, W.J. 1994. Privacy, confidentiality and privilege in psychotherapeutic relationships. *American Journal of Orthopsychiatry* 64(2): 180–193.
4. Wettstein, R. 1994. Confidentiality. *Review of Psychiatry* 13:343–364.
5. Bok, S. 1983. *Secrets: On the ethics of concealment and revelation*. New York: Pantheon Press, pp. 21–22.
6. American Medical Association. *Code of Medical Ethics*. Copyright 1996 American Medical Association, Chicago, Illinois.
7. Gutheil, T.G., Appelbaum, P.S. 1988. Confidentiality and privilege. In *Clinical Handbook of Psychiatry and the Law*. New York: McGraw-Hill Book Co., pp. 2–29.
8. Woodward, B. 1995. Medical record confidentiality and data collection: Current dilemmas. *Journal of Law Medicine and Ethics* 25(2–3):86–88.
9. Gostin, L.O. 1995. Genetic privacy. *Journal of Law Medicine and Ethics* 23: 320–330.
10. Bove, C.M., Fry, S., MacDonald, D.J. 1997. Pre-symptomatic and predisposition genetic testing: Ethical and social implications. *Seminars in Oncology Nursing* 13(2):135–140.

10

Information Disclosure:
Truth Telling

Objectives

The student should be able to:
- Discuss the health professional's role as a person who should maintain a patient's hope.
- Identify one major argument that traditionally has been advanced as to why patients should be protected from "bad news" and the ethical principles and reasoning that support this position.
- Identify major arguments that in recent years have been advanced as to why patients should be given information about their condition and the ethical principles and reasoning that support this position.
- Apply the six-step process of ethical analysis to truth-telling situations.
- Distinguish among the following notions: truth, deceit, lies, truth telling.
- Identify and discuss three instances in which a patient may be told a falsehood by a health professional.
- Define "placebo" and "placebo effect."
- Discuss possible benefits and harms of placebo use and the ethical principles that are important in analyzing placebo use from an ethics viewpoint.

New Terms and Ideas You Will Encounter in This Chapter

The professional's role to
   maintain hope
Benevolence
Information disclosure
Patient's right to information
Truth and falsehood

Deceit
Lies
Circularity
Placebos
Placebo effect

Topics in This Chapter Introduced in Earlier Chapters

Introduction

In the last chapter you were introduced to the value of trust and its role in confidentiality. In this chapter the focus is again on the idea of trust as it figures into truth-telling situations. In the next chapter trust is discussed in the context of informed consent.

In everyday life nothing is more central to a feeling of trust than assuming that others will be truthful in matters pertinent to our well-being. We assume that telling the truth is the right thing to do. Such action characterizes the honest person, and no one would question the moral value of honesty.

Therefore it may come as a surprise that giving direct and honest answers to patients has long been a topic of controversy in the health professions, particularly when bad news must be conveyed. Questions of truth telling are complex because there are other moral considerations within the relationship that may appear to conflict with the idea that "honesty is the best policy." One of these norms is the disposition or character trait of benevolence—that one should be the type of person who behaves toward others in a way that is not menacing or harmful to them.

To help our discussion along, consider the story of Andrew Gordon and Kim Segard.

THE STORY OF ANDREW GORDON AND KIM SEGARD

Andrew Gordon, a 43-year-old contractor, fell from a scaffold, fracturing his right tibia. A month earlier he had consulted his physician of 20 years, complaining of unusual fatigue. Tests revealed no abnormal findings, and Mr. Gordon returned to work. He believes he "blacked out" prior to the fall, but this is fuzzy to him.

Because the fracture is healing slowly, Mr. Gordon has been out of work for 3 weeks. The social worker, Kim Segard, has been visiting him often at Mr. Gordon's request. Mr. Gordon is discouraged about his slow recovery and worried about his wife and three children because he is self-employed, and every day away from work is a financial loss. Kim has been working to help Mr. Gordon arrange financial matters and provide support for the whole family. In the fourth week of hospitalization Mr. Gordon develops a fever during the night. The symptoms persist the next day so that all treatments must be canceled. Another series of tests is run, this time revealing a lymphosarcoma involving the bone, a type of cancer that is likely to be fatal within a year.

The physician, Lee Hammill, telephones Kim to report the diagnosis and its implications for treatment. He says he is quite certain that Mr. Gordon would not want to know that he has cancer. Kim asks Dr. Hammill why he has come to this conclusion, and he explains that Mr. Gordon once said of a friend who had died of cancer, "He stopped living as soon as he found out." The physician also tells Kim that he has spoken to Mrs. Gordon, who concurs with his judgment. He asks if Kim has had any discussion with Mr. or Mrs. Gordon that would provide insight into whether Mr. Gordon would want to know. Kim tries to think of something he may have said but is unable to recall any discussions that would clarify this difficult decision. Kim believes that both the Gordons have always confronted problems directly and honestly and says so. There is a pause. Lee Hammill puts an end to the conversation, replying, "Well, I've pretty much decided not to tell him. I think all in all it's better for him not to know."

Kim Segard goes on seeing Andrew Gordon. About ten days later he says to Kim, "You know, we have talked often, and I have come to trust your judgment. I'm grateful for the help you've given me and my family. You know I've tried to cooperate with the doctors and everyone, but I have a feeling that something funny is going on that I can't get at. My wife and Dr. Hammill are acting strange, and that is scaring me. I couldn't sleep all last night, and so I decided to ask you. I know you will level with me. . . . *Do I have cancer or some fatal illness?*"

Now that Kim Segard has been asked this question directly, what should she do? Should she tell Mr. Gordon? Not tell him? Take some other course of action?

Jot down your immediate response regarding what Kim should do:

In the history of health care there is a body of literature that would support not telling him and one supporting the truthful course of action. You will have an opportunity to think about your above response as you read the arguments against and for disclosure.

AN ARGUMENT AGAINST DISCLOSURE

The main argument advanced against disclosure of "bad news" is that the health professional's role is to *maintain the patient's hope,* and hope may be shattered by bad news. Do you agree that this is an important function you will have to assume? Yes _____ No _____

Throughout most of the history of Western health care the patient has been defined as the one who needs to be cared for, who has little knowledge of medical science, who suffers passively from a disease, and who brings herself or himself to the health care system much in the same way that a car is brought to an automobile mechanic. As Edward said to Dr. Reilly in T. S. Eliot's *The Cocktail Party,*

> I can no longer act for myself.
> Coming to see you—That's the last decision
> I was capable of making. I am in your hands.
> I cannot take any further responsibility.[1]

The patient's choice has been whether to follow the strong recommendations of the physician. Both character traits and duties are involved in this line of thinking. A *benevolent disposition* has been regarded as more important than an honest one, although both are extremely important. Which duties are involved in this type of situation? Name three:

1. _____
2. _____
3. _____

If you answered beneficence, nonmaleficence, and veracity you have correctly identified the duties that are consistent with being a benevolent or honest person.

As you may recall from our earlier discussions about duties, sometimes the idea of acting beneficently means acting independently of the patient's wishes. Such a way of acting is called _____ or _____. (The answer: paternalistic or parentalistic).

The arguments against disclosure of information have been based on paternalistic thinking. The health professional is privy to the awful truth of the inexorable progress of most diseases and decides what patients ought to be told based on an assessment of their welfare. Of course, such perceptions are heavily influenced by the professional's own concept of his or her role in the system and attitudes about sickness and death.

This portrays a relationship that is unequal and paternalistic but well intentioned. Honesty is sacrificed to benevolence to maintain a patient's trust. As you can easily discern, Dr. Hammill is being benevolent insofar as he judges his course of action to be in Mr. Gordon's best interests. Now Kim

Segard must make her own judgment about whether to act paternalistically or truthfully.

ARGUMENTS FAVORING DISCLOSURE

Today there is mounting pressure on the health professions from within their own ranks (as well as from lay people) to be more candid or honest with patients, especially concerning the health professional's own limitations. In the 1960s Elisabeth Kübler-Ross, a physician, spearheaded a revolutionary movement in the health care world by clarifying simple concepts about the dying process and making suggestions to improve care of the dying.[2] She was convinced that patients with fatal illnesses could handle the truth about that awesome knowledge and that therefore that knowledge ought not be swept under the rug delicately but rather dealt with honestly, carefully, and realistically. She cited many cases of people having come to terms with the meaning of death and dying for themselves and their loved ones because they knew the truth about their own condition and its prognosis. Today, thanks to Kübler-Ross and others like her, the topics of dying and death are not as taboo as they were a few years ago. In the wake of this new openness the idea that patients can handle difficult news and may even benefit from knowing has taken the health professionals down a new line of reasoning: the truth, rather than being a barrier to hope, may set the patient free. The AIDS epidemic has raised truth-telling questions and concerns to the forefront of health professionals' consciousness because if the patient does not know, he or she cannot be responsible for preventing the spread of the disease.

In this interpretation an honest disposition is at least as important as, and is not necessarily in conflict with, a benevolent one. Acting truthfully is consistent with acting beneficently. You cannot discern what is "best" for the patient by making decisions independently on his or her behalf. Caring entails sharing pertinent information: The best way to maintain trust is to share relevant information with patients but to do so in ways that will be supportive of them.

Truth telling involves a relationship between people, so that the issue of to tell or not to tell is merely a juncture in an ongoing personal and professional relationship with the one who asks the question. Underlying the bias toward greater disclosure of information is the conviction that if you convey the message that you still care and have the intention and ability to comfort, then it is possible to tell the truth and still maintain the patient's trust and hope. Benevolence is expressed *through* honesty rather than played off *against* it. Do you find these arguments compelling? Yes _____ No _____ Give examples to support your position.

_____

_____

Today an additional factor supporting more disclosure of information to patients is the understanding of patients' rights. It is believed that *patients have a right to information* about their conditions if they want this information. Recall from Chapter 3 that at least some rights correlate with duties. In this understanding of rights, if a person has a right to X, then it is someone's duty to give it to him or protect him in the possession of it. Who the someone is depends on their relationship. In today's consumer-oriented health care system, patients sometimes are called consumers. Accordingly a U.S. Presidential Advisory Commission on Consumer Protection and Quality in the Health Care Industry developed a Consumer Bill of Rights and Responsibilities to capture the challenges confronting everyone (see box, pp. 169 to 170). There are several similarities and differences in these guidelines to an older, widely used Patient's Bill of Rights developed by the American Hospital Association (see box, pp. 171 to 173). Compare the two documents.

In both documents there is an assumption that a patient has a right to the truth about his or her condition, and it is reasonable to believe that you, the health professional, do not have the prerogative of withholding it. There is a duty to share the information if the patient wishes this information, and withholding it can be viewed as a type of injury to the patient's trust. If information is withheld, it must be on the basis of other moral considerations deemed more compelling than the patient's right and your corresponding duty to disclose in a given situation.

Do you find the position that Mr. Gordon has a **right** to this information a compelling one?

Yes _____ No _____ Why? _____

Text continued on page 174

CONSUMER BILL OF RIGHTS AND RESPONSIBILITIES

Consumer Rights

I. *Information Disclosure*
   Consumers have the right to receive accurate, easily understood information and some require assistance in making informed health care decisions about their health plans, professionals, and facilities.

II. *Choice of Providers and Plans*
   Consumers have the right to a choice of health care providers that is sufficient to ensure access to appropriate high-quality health care.

III. *Access to Emergency Services*
   Consumers have the right to access emergency health care services when and where the need arises.

IV. *Participation in Treatment Decisions*
   Consumers have the right and responsibility to fully participate in all decisions related to their health care. Consumers who are unable to fully participate in treatment decisions have the right to be represented by parents, guardians, family members, or other conservators.

V. *Respect and Nondiscrimination*
   Consumers have the right to considerate, respectful care from all members of the health care system at all times and under all circumstances. An environment of mutual respect is essential to maintain a quality health care system.
   Consumers must not be discriminated against in the delivery of health care services.
   Consumers who are eligible for coverage under the terms and conditions of a health plan or program or as required by law must not be discriminated against in marketing and enrollment practices based on race, ethnicity, national origin, religion, sex, age, mental or physical disability, sexual orientation, genetic information, or source of payment.

VI. *Confidentiality of Health Information*
   Consumers have the right to communicate with health care providers in confidence and to have the confidentiality of their individually identifiable health care information protected. Consumers also have the right to review and copy their own medical records and request amendments to their records.

VII. *Complaints and Appeals*
   All consumers have the right to a fair and efficient process for resolving differences with their health plans, health care providers, and the institutions that serve them, including a rigorous system of internal review and an independent system of external review.

Box continued on following page

CONSUMER BILL OF RIGHTS AND RESPONSIBILITIES *Continued*

Consumer Responsibilities

In a health care system that protects consumers' rights, it is reasonable to expect and encourage consumers to assume reasonable responsibilities.

1. Take responsibility for maximizing healthy habits, such as exercising, not smoking, and eating a healthy diet.
2. Become involved in specific health care decisions.
3. Work collaboratively with health care providers in developing and carrying out agreed-upon treatment plans.
4. Disclose relevant information and clearly communicate wants and needs.
5. Use the health plan's internal complaint and appeal processes to address concerns that may arise.
6. Avoid knowingly spreading disease.
7. Recognize the reality of risks and limits of the science of medical care and the human fallibility of the health care professional.
8. Be aware of a health care provider's obligation to be reasonably efficient and equitable in providing care to other patients and the community.
9. Become knowledgeable about his or her health plan coverage and health plan options (when available) including all covered benefits, limitations, and exclusions, rules regarding use of network providers, coverage and referral rules, appropriate processes to secure additional information, and the process to appeal coverage decisions.
10. Show respect for other patients and health workers.
11. Make a good-faith effort to meet financial obligations.
12. Abide by administrative and operational procedures of health plans, health care providers, and government health benefit programs.
13. Report wrongdoing and fraud to appropriate resources or legal authorities.

Summary of the *Consumer Bill of Rights and Responsibilities: Report to the President of the United States* prepared by the Advisory Commission on Consumer Protection and Quality in the Health Care Industry, November 1997. U.S. Government Printing Office.

A PATIENT'S BILL OF RIGHTS

Introduction

Effective health care requires collaboration between patients and physicians and other health care professionals. Open and honest communication, respect for personal and professional values, and sensitivity to differences are integral to optimal patient care. As the setting for the provision of health services, hospitals must provide a foundation for understanding and respecting the rights and responsibilities of patients, their families, physicians, and other caregivers. Hospitals must ensure a health care ethic that respects the role of patients in decision making about treatment choices and other aspects of their care. Hospitals must be sensitive to cultural, racial, linguistic, religious, age, gender, and other differences as well as the needs of persons with disabilities.

The American Hospital Association presents *A Patient's Bill of Rights* with the expectation that it will contribute to more effective patient care and be supported by the hospital on behalf of the institution, its medical staff, employees, and patients. The American Hospital Association encourages health care institutions to tailor this bill of rights to their patient community by translating and/or simplifying the language of this bill of rights as may be necessary to ensure that patients and their families understand their rights and responsibilities.

Bill of Rights*

1. The patient has the right to considerate and respectful care.

2. The patient has the right to and is encouraged to obtain from physicians and other direct caregivers relevant, current, and understandable information concerning diagnosis, treatment, and prognosis.

   Except in emergencies when the patient lacks decision-making capacity and the need for treatment is urgent, the patient is entitled to the opportunity to discuss and request information related to the specific procedures and/or treatments, the risks involved, the possible length of recuperation, and the medically reasonable alternatives and their accompanying risks and benefits.

   Patients have the right to know the identity of physicians, nurses, and others involved in their care, as well as when those involved are students, residents, or other trainees. The patient also has the right to know the immediate and long-term financial implications of treatment choices, insofar as they are known.

3. The patient has the right to make decisions about the plan of care prior to and during the course of treatment and to refuse a recommended treatment or plan of care to the extent permitted by law and hospital policy and to be informed of the medical consequences of this action. In case of such refusal, the patient is entitled to other appropriate care and services that the hospital provides or transfer to another hospital. The hospital should notify patients of any policy that might affect patient choice within the institution.

---

*These rights can be exercised on the patient's behalf by a designated surrogate or proxy decision maker if the patient lacks decision-making capacity, is legally incompetent, or is a minor.

Box continued on following page

A PATIENT'S BILL OF RIGHTS *Continued*

4. The patient has the right to have an advance directive (such as a living will, health care proxy, or durable power of attorney for health care) concerning treatment or designating a surrogate decision maker with the expectation that the hospital will honor the intent of that directive to the extent permitted by law and hospital policy.

   Health care institutions must advise patients of their rights under state law and hospital policy to make informed medical choices, ask if the patient has an advance directive, and include that information in patient records. The patient has the right to timely information about hospital policy that may limit its ability to implement fully a legally valid advance directive.

5. The patient has the right to every consideration of privacy. Case discussion, consultation, examination, and treatment should be conducted so as to protect each patient's privacy.

6. The patient has the right to expect that all communications and records pertaining to his/her care will be treated as confidential by the hospital, except in cases such as suspected abuse and public health hazards when reporting is permitted or required by law. The patient has the right to expect that the hospital will emphasize the confidentiality of this information when it releases it to any other parties entitled to review information in these records.

7. The patient has the right to review the records pertaining to his/her medical care and to have the information explained or interpreted as necessary, except when restricted by law.

8. The patient has the right to expect that, within its capacity and policies, a hospital will make reasonable response to the request of a patient for appropriate and medically indicated care and services. The hospital must provide evaluation, service, and/or referral as indicated by the urgency of the case. When medically appropriate and legally permissible, or when a patient has so requested, a patient may be transferred to another facility. The institution to which the patient is to be trasferred must first have accepted the patient for transfer. The patient must also have the benefit of complete information and explanation concerning the need for, risks, benefits, and alternatives to such a transfer.

9. The patient has the right to ask and be informed of the existence of business relationships among the hospital, educational institutions, other health care providers, or payers that may influence the patient's treatment and care.

10. The patient has the right to consent to or decline to participate in proposed research studies or human experimentation affecting care and treatment or requiring direct patient involvement, and to have those studies fully explained prior to consent. A patient who declines to participate in research or experimentation is entitled to the most effective care that the hospital can otherwise provide.

A PATIENT'S BILL OF RIGHTS *Continued*

11. The patient has the right to expect reasonable continuity of care when appropriate and to be informed by physicians and other caregivers of available and realistic patient care options when hospital care is no longer appropriate.

12. The patient has the right to be informed of hospital policies and practices that relate to patient care, treatment, and responsibilities. The patient has the right to be informed of available resources for resolving disputes, grievances, and conflicts, such as ethics committees, patient representatives, or other mechanisms available in the institution. The patient has the right to be informed of the hospital's charges for services and available payment methods.

The collaborative nature of health care requires that patients, or their families/surrogates, participate in their care. The effectiveness of care and patient satisfaction with the course of treatment depend, in part, on the patient fulfilling certain responsibilities. Patients are responsible for providing information about past illnesses, hospitalizations, medications, and other matters related to health status. To participate effectively in decision making, patients must be encouraged to take responsibility for requesting additional information or clarification about their health status or treatment when they do not fully understand information and instructions. Patients are also responsible for ensuring that the health care institution has a copy of their written advance directive if they have one. Patients are responsible for informing their physicians and other caregivers if they anticipate problems in following prescribed treatment.

Patients should also be aware of the hospital's obligation to be reasonably efficient and equitable in providing care to other patients and the community. The hospital's rules and regulations are designed to help the hospital meet this obligation. Patients and their families are responsible for making reasonable accommodations to the needs of the hospital, other patients, medical staff, and hospital employees. Patients are responsible for providing necessary information for insurance claims and for working with the hospital to make payment arrangements, when necessary.

A person's health depends on much more than health care services. Patients are responsible for recognizing the impact of their life-style on their personal health.

Conclusion

Hospitals have many functions to perform, including the enhancement of health status, health promotion, and the prevention and treatment of injury and disease; the immediate and ongoing care and rehabilitation of patients; the education of health professionals, patients, and the community; and research. All these activities must be conducted with an overriding concern for the values and dignity of patients.

APPLYING THE SIX-STEP PROCESS OF DECISION MAKING

Step 1: Gather Relevant Information

Kim's benevolence and honesty and the corresponding duties of benefi-cence and veracity support her attempt to assess Mr. Gordon's request accurately. It is possible that Mr. Gordon is asking Kim this question because he wants Kim to reassure him that he does not have a fatal illness. It is also possible that during the long weeks of hospitalization Andrew Gordon has developed a new attitude about his own life and death and truly does want to know.

It is important to be sensitive to the implicit, unspoken messages that are contained in language. This is true of all verbal communications between persons. Mr. Gordon here is expressing a nameless fear with the question, "Do I have cancer?" His fear is undoubtedly related to the idea of fatal illness, but often in such cases anxiety is heightened by the feelings of helplessness and insecurity that arise when an intelligent person who was strong and self-sufficient finds himself in a situation in which he doubts the sincerity of those in whom he has had the greatest trust (his wife and physician). Here we see one of the greatest risks of the attitude of benevolence not coupled with honesty: In assuming the responsibility for protecting a patient from the knowledge of his disease, we cannot protect him from the disease and its consequences and may, in fact, heighten his psychological torment by making him feel deceived by those charged with his care.

Mr. Gordon's real question may concern the extent of Kim's (and the health professions') commitment to him. He may be asking beyond "Do I have cancer?" to "If I have cancer will you still care for me?" Often the diagnosis of a fatal or disabling chronic disease causes professionals to withdraw from contact with the afflicted person, and patients can sense this shift in attitude, however subtle or covert. Initially the health professional's reaction may be one of horror, embarrassment, or nervousness. The patient, responding to these changes, will become more anxious and may need support and comfort from health professionals as much or more than he needs therapeutic measures aimed at relieving his symptoms. At such times the therapeutic encounters in which the health professionals are involved must become the vehicle for such comfort. Regularly scheduled appointments, active gestures of caring, and just simply being there can assure the patient that the health professional, and by implication all the powers of the healing professions, will not abandon him.

In short, the first important step in Kim's assessment of this situation is to *gather the relevant information* by gaining a better understanding of what Mr. Gordon is asking.

I have listed some types of information I think are relevant. What other types of information would you want to have before proceeding in this situation? List them here.

_____

_____

Step 2: Identify the Type of Ethical Problem

In this situation Kim is faced with ethical distress. She thinks Mr. Gordon should have the information. Indeed a central problem for Kim—and for health professionals other than physicians—specifically has to do with professional relationships. Nurses, chaplains, technologists, technicians, dietitians, pharmacists, social workers, and others may find themselves in the difficult position of being caught in the middle between the wishes of the physicians and their own assessment of the best interests of the patient.

The structure of the health care system, as it has developed throughout history, has been characterized by hierarchical relationships. All but physicians in this traditional hierarchy have been assigned the role to act in full accordance with the best judgment of the physician. They seldom have authority to determine a course of action independent of a physician's orders, although they often spend a great deal more time with patients than physicians do and may develop closer personal relationships. The rationale in the traditional medical model was that the physician holds the greatest amount of concrete biomedical information, so therefore she or he was the person best able to coordinate necessary procedures and to make major therapy decisions, which were then implemented through the skills of other health professionals. Today that model is being altered somewhat because there are more types of prefessionals who serve as points of entry into the health care system and because of the greater sophistication of many team members. A well-coordinated effort on behalf of the patient makes the most efficient use of resources, time, and energy and supports the patient's attitude of trust toward those entrusted with his or her care. But it appears in Kim's situation that both she and Dr. Hammill assume that the physician has the authority to decide whether and what information should be shared with Mr. Gordon.

(NOTE: If you have had difficulty identifying the types of problems, go back and review Chapter 4 before proceeding.)

Step 3: Determine the Ethics Approach to Be Used

This step is designed to encourage you to again reflect consciously on your basic ethical approach to complex problems, problems such as those illustrated by the story of Mr. Gordon. You probably have recognized that my heavy reliance on the duties and rights that come into conflict in this story places me within the _____ framework or approach to this issue. It is not surprising that I am drawn to this deontological approach, as much of the traditional health care approach to ethical problems relies on an understanding of our various duties, commitments, rights, or loyalties. Do you also find yourself thinking as a deontologist about this problem?

A rights-governed approach would require that the rights of the several parties involved be identified and weighed. I have mentioned one important right that Mr. Gordon has as a patient, the right to information, and you have had an opportunity to review some others in the AHA Patient's Bill of Rights. What rights does Dr. Hammill have in this situation? What rights does Kim Segard have?

If you depend on neither duties nor rights, your approach is less means oriented than ends oriented. The ends-oriented or consequences-oriented approach you learned is _teleology_, the most common form of which is _____. (If you did not answer "utilitarianism," you should go back and review the theories in Chapter 3 again.) Which consequences are relevant for our consideration in the story of Mr. Gordon? Which ones would weigh the most heavily? Why? _____

_____

_____

Once you have identified the relevant duties, rights, and consequences and have determined the approach you will use, you are able to determine an _ideal_ course of action. This ideal course should also be guided by character traits that dispose you to want to do what your compassion and integrity counsel you to do. Without such help you may choose to take a course that fails to be the best for Mr. Gordon and his family as persons.

As we live in a less than perfect world, however, you must now begin the arduous practical task of identifying the several alternatives that are most likely to enable you to act in accordance with your analysis and your disposition to do what is best for them.

Step 4: Explore the Practical Alternatives

In the situation of Mr. Gordon, seemingly good rapport exists between the physician and social worker. Dr. Hammill expresses concern regarding Mr. Gordon's psychological state and has given it much thought before making the decision not to inform him of the diagnosis. This decision has been reached "for his own good," and the information for its support has come not only from the patient and the patient's wife but also to some extent from the social worker, Kim Segard. As the doctor did take the trouble to call Kim and ask if the patient had conveyed any information to her that might temper the interpretation of his statement concerning his feeling about people with cancer, it seems that the door is open for Kim to contact Dr. Hammill regarding Mr. Gordon's question. Thus the fourth step in Kim's process of moral judgment and action may well be to decide to telephone the physician at once. In this action, Kim is fulfilling her professional loyalty to the physician in a way that is likely to benefit the patient as well. But this solution works only in a setting of good communication and mutual respect between the various members of the health care team and in situations in which the patient clearly can trust that Kim and others have his or her best interests at the center of their decision making.

Kim is still faced with the decision about what to say to Andrew Gordon when the question is first posed. What do you think you would say?

You could say, "I don't know all the results of your tests, but I can see you are really worried about it. Why don't you ask the doctor about it when he comes by later today?" or, even, "Shall I speak to Dr. Hammill and tell him that you are concerned about your progress?" The decision you make about how to answer the question does not end with that answer but requires the fifth step of ethical analysis—completion of the action. In this case the action is to contact Dr. Hammill as soon as possible. Assurance that the physician will respond wisely to this turn of events helps to determine your own course of action.

The caught-in-the-middle experience of ethical distress can sometimes be alleviated if you keep your eyes and ears open to earlier signs of the types of worries a patient has. Because you may spend long, predictable periods of time with a patient, he or she is likely to be able to pick up subtle messages about your uncertainty and anxiety. For example, Mr. Gordon has probably not made a conscious decision that "If I have cancer, I want to know about it." Clearly he is suffering from this insecurity, and you or another health professional might have noticed this in earlier interactions with him. These impressions could be communicated to the physician and the issue reevaluated *before* the actual question is posed.

Indeed you should work closely with the physician throughout the course of a patient's care and keep communications open among physician, patient, other significant people, and yourself. For example, at the time of the telephone call Kim made, you could:

1. Advise the physician you will tell Mr. Gordon his diagnosis if Mr. Gordon should ask directly. You will then know what to expect from the physician when it happens, or the conversation may give you

some guidelines about how you two professionals can best work together and also prepare other professional colleagues to be ready for
such a question.
2. Tell the physician you would like to talk to Mrs. Gordon and report
back to the physician or meet with the two of them.
3. Tell the physician you will not tell Mr. Gordon his diagnosis or prognosis but will inform the physician of any pertinent questions or comments made by the Gordons.
4. Suggest that Dr. Hammill talk to the nurse or to any other person
whom you know to be close to Mr. Gordon or who may have insight
into how to proceed.
5. Actively support the physician in his attempt to discover Mr. Gordon's wishes. This may lead to further discussion between you,
putting you more on a basis of mutual trust and respect.
6. Ask the physician why he thinks Mrs. Gordon concurred or if Mrs.
Gordon initiated the idea.

Or, before seeing Mr. Gordon again, you could:

1. Think through possible conditions under which you will tell Mr. Gordon that he has cancer.
2. Talk to Mrs. Gordon.
3. Talk to the nurse or others who may know how Mr. Gordon may react.

If the situation were different and you (or any health professional) felt
the physician was unresponsive to the patient's needs or was not open to
communication of this sort from others, then the problem is much more difficult. If the physician is not acting in a way that seems to be furthering the
patient's well-being, you could ask the ethics committee or ethics consultant
in the institution to help. Such resources increasingly are available and have
as their goal the resolution of ethical problems such as the one this social
worker is facing.

If all these alternatives fail, a last resort alternative is that you may decide to tell the patient and risk the personal consequences. In many settings
these consequences could range from a simple reprimand all the way to the
loss of your job.

Now that you have read *my* list of ideas about the options, add some
more of your own if you have them: _____

_____

_____

Step 5: Complete the Action

Whatever you have decided to do, you now need the courage to do it.
The hardest case scenario is if you have to break faith with the physician.
This should be considered only when:

1. You are convinced the patient is requesting a direct answer about diagnosis or prognosis, and
2. You believe that the patient's request can be honored *only* by your personally delivering that information, and
3. You feel obligated to be the one to share the information in spite of the physician's request that it not be shared.

Step 6: Evaluate the Process and Outcome

When you have completed the action, have you carried out your professional responsibility? If upon reviewing your action you realize it followed the most thorough and careful ethical analysis that you are able to exercise in this situation, you can rest assured that you have given everyone involved your best effort. Checking out your thinking with colleagues can further help you make an accurate assessment.

TRUTH, TRUTH TELLING, AND DECEIT

We have been discussing Mr. Gordon's predicament as a truth-telling issue, but we have not really discussed the basic concepts involved: truth, falsehood, deceit, lies, truth telling. To do so was not crucial for your thinking to this point, but it will be important for the next section on placebos. Thus I'll take a minute to do that now.

Truth is one of those wonderfully rich concepts in philosophy that is easiest to understand by talking about it in relationship to its opposite. Of course, in philosophy there are whole theories of truth: a coherence theory, a correspondence theory, a performative one, and a pragmatic theory, to name some, each of which tries to place truth within the world of our concepts. For our purposes we will take the more common everyday approach and compare it with its opposite. What is a *falsehood?*

If you answered, "an untruth," you are correct, but more explanation is required to avoid the problem that philosophers call *circularity*, or *circular reasoning* (e.g., a truth is the opposite of an untruth, and an untruth is the opposite of a truth).

A more helpful way to think about an untruth or falsehood is to consider how it functions in our everyday life. When someone utters a falsehood, it is either out of not having accurate information or out of an intent to deceive the listener. When a person does not have the accurate information, we judge the person to be ignorant or even negligent (if it is information another has a reasonable expectation of the person in question knowing). If the intent is to deceive, we say that the person is *lying*.

> ## A LIE IS AN INTENT TO DECEIVE.

In Mr. Gordon's situation, he was not getting information about his condition from his physician. Was Dr. Hammill ignorant, negligent, or intending to deceive?_____

_____

_____

From what we know I believe Dr. Hammill intended to deceive Mr. Gordon by neglecting to tell him his condition. Although we usually do not talk about the withholding of information as lying, the neglect to intervene when one is morally obligated to do so can be a form of lying. This has the confusing term, "an act of omission."

This brings us to our next practical point regarding these concepts. Information-sharing discussions in the health professions context are about uttering true statements or, as we usually call it, truth telling. Our concern is about the converse, what we might call falsehood telling. The telling of a falsehood from ignorance may entail carelessness or incompetence. The intent to deceive by knowingly giving false information or withholding true information does not entail carelessness or incompetence. And so we must explore the situation further to know how to judge Dr. Hammill's falsehood. As we have seen, Dr. Hammill decided to deceive Mr. Gordon on the basis of a paternalistic posture toward this patient. Kim Segard is not at all convinced that Mr. Gordon is actually benefiting from this deception. One should think of information as power to be used or abused by the moral agent. Therefore, whenever information is being withheld or distorted, you must begin your assessment by ascertaining why this is occurring.

I hope that this brief background regarding the concepts related to truths and falsehoods will help you to examine your own conduct when you are confronted with challenging situations. To complete this chapter I want to draw your attention to an important related idea in health care—placebos.

PLACEBOS: A SPECIAL CASE OF INFORMATION DISCLOSURE

The issue of *placebo* use has received some attention from psychiatrists and ethicists, but most literature on placebos has been directed toward physicians. Little research has been done concerning the role of health professionals and the use of placebo medications and procedures, and yet nurses and pharmacists, in particular, play a direct and essential part in this particular form of deception in health care practice. To think clearly about the ethical problems that may arise in such a situation it is important to understand the physician's role in prescribing a placebo and some of the history and psychology of the placebo response.

Placebo comes from the Latin word meaning "I shall please." It can be defined as any therapeutic procedure (or component of one) that is given for a condition on which it has no known pharmacologic effect. A pure placebo is a preparation of an inert substance that is not known to have any pharmacologic effect. An impure placebo is an active drug given for its psychological effect even though it has no known effect on the disorder in question, such as an antibiotic for a common cold or other viral infection. Administering this type of placebo carries the risk of real side effects, as well as the interpersonal and professional risks we will discuss in regard to pure placebos.

Physicians rarely give pure placebos, such as sugar pills or saline injections, but when they do, serious ethical issues need to be considered. One important aspect of the practice of giving placebos is what is called the placebo effect. Virtually all treatments (and some diagnostic studies as well) have positive effects for some patients over and above the specific effects of their pharmacologic mechanisms. Beecher published the classic study in 1955 showing that placebos are effective in treating pain in 35% of patients, regardless of the source of pain or clinical condition of the patient.[3] Modern neuropharmacology research has discovered that the brain produces its own chemicals, which can act as analgesics and relaxants. These chemicals, called endorphins, seem to work better for some people than for others, which may explain scientifically why some people are placebo reactors and others are not. A common error made by health professionals has been the assumption that a symptom (for example, pain) successfully treated by a placebo is therefore not real or "only psychological." The discovery of endorphins gives us a scientific way of understanding some of the powerful physiological effects of placebos.

The placebo effect may be partly responsible for the success of ancient remedies given by shamans or medicine men. Some of these remedies contained pharmacologically active agents, but others did not, and much of the healer's work consisted of rituals and symbols. The fact that the medicine men were often successful is a tribute to the power of the physician-patient relationship or the therapeutic partnership.

Modern examples of the placebo effect are the effects of suggestion in decreasing stomach acid in ulcer patients, alleviating bronchospasm in asthma, and lowering blood pressure. The phenomenon of the placebo effect is widespread and powerful enough so that no research trials of new medications or even surgical procedures are considered truly rigorous unless the element of suggestion has been effectively eliminated, as in randomized double-blind clinical trials.

Some philosophers oppose the use of true placebos in health care because they see it as an example of deception or outright lying.[4] We have considered the problem of lying to patients in regard to the disclosure of serious or terminal disease. Are there significant differences in the area of placebo use that might justify deception? Yes _____ No _____ Why?

_____

_____

A utilitarian approach to thinking about the use of placebos would suggest that one must weigh positive effects against the possible negative ones that could result from placebo therapy. What do you think are some of the potential harmful consequences?

1. _____

2. _____

3. _____

Now that you have listed some I will briefly review a few that often are suggested:

Loss of trust in the therapeutic relationship is viewed as one of the major risks of placebo use. Such deception preempts the patient's capacity to share in the responsibility for his or her health. Philosophers have noted that allowing deception in our professional and private relationships tends to diminish the overall quality of those relationships.

Melmon and Morelli point out another danger, that of inadequate diagnosis.[5] If a physician is too quick to use a placebo for treating a patient's aches and pains, a potentially serious and treatable medical disorder may be overlooked. Thus it is important that a thorough medical and psychological evaluation be made if the use of the placebo therapy is to be considered.

Much of the harm attributed to placebo use comes when it is given without respect for the patient as a person. Physicians may prescribe placebos inappropriately: They may use them to prove patients wrong when they feel too angry to give the patient real medication, to punish problem patients, or to release staff frustrations.[6] Health professionals find it difficult to respect patients who respond to placebos because of our emphasis on mechanistic physiological explanations. Many health professionals feel that a patient's positive response to a placebo indicates that the symptom is not real, even though this has been disproved by many studies like Beecher's and by the recent discovery of endorphins. A good response to placebos does not indicate that the patient is hypochondriacal. Patients in perfect mental health with real pain and illness may respond to placebos.[7] In fact, cooperative patients who have stable relationships with their caregivers are more likely to respond well to placebos than are the more difficult or less cooperative patients. Thus these are significant risks that ought always to be kept in mind, but it seems unwise to rule out the possibility of placebo use completely. We are beginning to learn more about the therapeutic powers (psychological

and chemical) of the mind, but we must also remember that we live in a society that has become dependent on pills and potions—symbolically and actually. Compassion allows us to use placebos in situations where a patient
may be respectfully benefited and where that patient is likely to be unable
to produce the desired effect without the symbol of the medication or other
medical procedure.

SUMMARY

The story of Mr. Gordon is just one example of the ethical problems involved in the issue of truth telling. Our discussion is intended to stimulate
your thoughts on the subject and not to cover all the possible situations you
are likely to encounter. Here, as in the other issues in this section of the
book, the decision about what to do is influenced by what is deemed necessary for maintaining the patient's trust and to acknowledge his or her dignity
as a human being. The six-step process will assist you in proceeding to a decision and acting on it. But the situation may require action in the face of
seemingly unresolvable conflict or may carry the potential of dire personal
consequences. At such moments the dispositions of honesty, benevolence,
and courage support you in persevering in what you judge to be the most appropriate of the options available. The special case of placebo use continues
to provide an illustration of how complex the truth-telling issues can become. As you develop in your professional role, you will have ample opportunity for reflection and thoughtful action around these issues.

Questions for Thought and Discussion

1. Immanuel Kant, a philosopher of the formalist school, has declared,
   "The duty of being truthful . . . is unconditional. To be truthful in all de-
   clarations, . . . is a sacred and absolutely commanding decree of reason,
   limited by no expediency."[8]

   In contrast, Nicolai Hartmann, a contemporary philosopher, has
   maintained that in health care practice the health professional is sometimes required to tell the "necessary lie" to avoid inflicting great harm on
   the patient.[9] Describe where you are on this continuum and why. Give
   examples from health care to support your position.

2. You have been receiving placebos.

   a. What would be your initial response to your physician if she informed
      you the medication that was relieving your severe stomach pains was
      a sugar capsule?

   b. Suppose that your physician feels obliged to tell you about the placebo
      used to relieve your stomach problems. How might she disclose this

information in a way that affirms the caring aspects of her relationship with you?

3. It has been maintained that patients have a right to the information about their conditions. But what happens when the diagnosis reveals a *genetic* disorder that can have harmful effects on the children? Should the spouse automatically be told? The children? Other relatives? Who is "the patient" in such situations?

4. Is there a right *not* to know the truth? Under what, if any, conditions might such a right be argued?

References

1. From *The Cocktail Party*, copyright 1950 by T.S. Eliot; renewed 1978 by Esme Válerie Eliot. Reprinted by permission of Harcourt, Brace Jovanovich, Inc.
2. Kübler-Ross, E. 1969. *On Death and Dying*. New York: Macmillan.
3. Beecher, H.K. 1955. The powerful placebo. *Journal of the American Medical Association* 159:1602–1606.
4. Bok, S. 1978. *Lying: Moral Choice in Public and Private Life*. New York: Pantheon Books, p. 11.
5. Melmon, K.L., Morelli, H.F. 1972. *Clinical Pharmacology: Basic Principles in Therapeutics*. New York: Macmillan, pp. 558–565.
6. *Ibid*. p. 565.
7. Dyer, A.R. 1988. *Ethics and Psychiatry: Toward Professional Definition*. Washington, DC: American Psychiatric Association Press, pp. 80–82.
8. Kant, I. In *Lectures on Ethics* (translated by Louis Infield). 1963. New York: Harper & Row, pp. 147–154.
9. Hartmann, N. 1932. *Ethics*. New York: Humanities Press, p. 282.

11

Informed Consent

Objectives

The student should be able to:
- Describe and distinguish between several basic ethical and legal concepts in the doctrine of informed consent.
- Identify the type of claim a patient's right to autonomy places on the health professional.
- Describe the contractual nature of informed consent.
- Discuss two major challenges that affect the success of the informed consent process.
- Describe three approaches to determining the standard for judging that a patient or client has been informed.
- Distinguish "general consent" from "special consent" documents.
- Differentiate between the never competent and once competent patient or client, and the challenges posed by each in regard to informed consent.
- Identify four types of advance directives.
- Compare informed consent as it is used in health care practice and in human studies research.
- Distinguish between "therapeutic research" and "nontherapeutic research."

New Terms and Ideas You Will Encounter in This Chapter

Informed consent
Battery (legal)
Disclosure (legal)
Fiduciary relationship (legal)
Contract (legal)
Disclosure standards
General consent
Special consent

Voluntariness
Mental competence or incompetence
Mental capacitation or incapacitation
Never competent or capacitated
Once competent or capacitated
Surrogate proxy consent
Best interests standard
Substituted judgment standard

Guardian (legal)
Advance directives
Therapeutic research

Nontherapeutic research
Institutional review board (IRB)

Topics in This Chapter Introduced in Earlier Chapters

TOPIC	INTRODUCED IN	DISCUSSED IN THIS CHAPTER ON
Rights, moral	Chapter 3	Page 190
Right to self-determination	Chapter 3	Page 190
Autonomy	Chapter 3	Pages 190, 192, 194
Beneficence	Chapter 3	Page 191
Nonmaleficence	Chapter 3	Page 191
Trust	Chapter 2	Page 190
Deontological approach	Chapter 3	Page 201

Introduction

One important avenue to your success as a professional is to perfect the communication, listening, and interpretive skills required to honor the tenets of the doctrine of *informed consent*, one of the cornerstones of the current U.S. and Canadian health care systems. Although the doctrine is the most formalized in these countries, it is an important concept in most Western health care systems. Whether engaging with patients, clients, or research subjects, basic principles of respect for the person undergird informed consent. To inform your thinking as you read this chapter, consider the story of Jason F and Faye N:

INFORMED CONSENT AND JASON F'S HIV TEST RESULTS

Jason F, a 34-year-old cross-country truck driver, came to the emergency room of his hometown hospital because of "kidney problems" and dehydration. When Faye N, the nurse practitioner, took his history, she noted that Jason had the scars of an active IV drug user. When she asked him about it, he admitted to "shooting up to cut the boredom" of his frequent cross-country jaunts.

Faye stated that Jason should have an HIV antibody test because it would be crucial to his diagnosis and treatment. When Jason expressed concern about confidentiality, the nurse practitioner told him that such test results were carefully guarded. In fact, only the patient, she, the attending physician, and the laboratory technician would know the test was being done. He said he would do it if it would help him get rid of his kidney infection, but when she presented him with the consent form, he said, "You got a noose around my neck. I know I gotta sign this thing to get treated." The test was performed. He was given some medications for his acute symptoms, and with that Jason left the emergency room with a follow-up appointment set for two weeks later.

Ten days later Jason reappeared in the emergency room with dysuria and peripheral edema in both legs. He was admitted to the hospital with a diagnosis of hypertension and life-threatening acute renal failure. His HIV antibody result had come back positive, but Jason had not been informed of this. When a staff nurse mentioned this to him, he became enraged. He called for Faye, who came up to the unit to see him. He claimed he had never been told the results would be placed in his medical record and, in fact, had been led to believe only three people besides himself would ever know the test results.

Faye said she was sorry that he had learned about the test results in this way but that she had explained everything to him before he signed the consent form. She said she believed any patient should know that the results would have to be recorded in the medical record. "You said they would be 'carefully guarded,'" he retorted. "Is this your idea of 'careful?'" She replied that when she said they would be carefully guarded she meant that no one among the professional staff who saw them would talk about it to anyone who should not have access to this sensitive information.

Before you continue, take a minute to jot down your own response to this situation in regard to Faye's role. Did she fulfill her legal and ethical obligation to obtain informed consent from Jason? What were the strengths of her approach in this situation? Could she have done a better job of obtaining informed consent?

Given your reading so far, what other ethical issues does this story raise?

_____

_____

_____

You will have an opportunity to revisit their situation as you study this chapter. You can begin to assess it by comparing it with any you may have had, although the details probably will be quite different.

Have you ever given your "informed consent" for a treatment or diagnostic intervention or for participation as a research subject? Yes_____ No_____. Did someone explain to you what was going to happen? Yes_____ No_____. Did you have to fill out a form? Yes_____ No_____ I cannot remember _____. If you completed a form, jot down here what you remember about it. (What did it say? Could you understand it easily? Did you have to sign your name? Was there someone on hand to answer questions you may have had at the time or a telephone number of where to reach someone later? Did reading and signing the form make you feel more reassured about what you were about to experience?)

_____

_____

_____

Now that you have a story to refer to and have considered your own experience if any, you are ready to read on about informed consent in general.

INFORMED CONSENT IN HEALTH CARE DECISIONS

Informed consent is founded on basic legal-ethical principles, entails a process of decision making, and is a procedure. The idea is that you can perform your professional tasks better and in a morally defensible way by bringing the person's informed preferences into your plans.

An example of an informed consent document (Fig. 11–1) spells out how the health professional intends to use specific diagnostic or treatment

---

MEDICAL RECORD	REQUEST FOR ADMINISTRATION OF ANESTHESIA AND FOR PERFORMANCE OF OPERATIONS AND OTHER PROCEDURES

A. IDENTIFICATION

1. OPERATION OR PROCEDURE

B. STATEMENT OF REQUEST

1. The nature and purpose of the operation or procedure, possible alternative methods of treatment, the risks involved, and the possibility of complications have been fully explained to me. I acknowledge that no guarantees have been made to me concerning the results of the operation or procedure. I understand the nature of the operation or procedure to be_____

(Description of operation or procedure in layman's language)

2. I request the performance of the above-named operation or procedure and of such additional operations or procedures as are found to be necessary or desirable, in the judgment of the professional staff of the below-named medical facility, during the course of the above-named operation or procedure.

3. I request the administration of such anesthesia as may be considered necessary or advisable in the judgment of the professional staff of the below-named medical facility.

4. Exceptions to surgery or anesthesia, if any, are:_____

(If "none", so state)

5. I request the disposal by authorities of the below-named medical facility of any tissues or parts which it may be necessary to remove.

6. I understand that photographs and movies may be taken of this operation, and that they may be viewed by various personnel undergoing training or indoctrination at this or other facilities. I consent to the taking of such pictures and observation of the operation by authorized personnel, subject to the following conditions:

    a. The name of the patient and his/her family is not used to identify said pictures.

    b. Said pictures be used only for purposes of medical study or research.

(Cross out any parts above which are not appropriate)

C. SIGNATURES   *(Appropriate items in Parts A and B must be completed before signing)*

1. COUNSELING PHYSICIAN: I have counseled this patient as to the nature of the proposed procedure(s), attendant risks involved, and expected results, as described above.

_____
(Signature of Counseling Physician)

2. PATIENT: I understand the nature of the proposed procedure(s), attendant risks involved, and expected results, as described above, and hereby request such procedure(s) be performed.

_____   _____
(Signature of Witness, excluding members of operating team)   (Signature of Patient)   (Date & Time)

3. SPONSOR OR GUARDIAN: (When patient is a minor or unable to give consent) I,_____ sponsor/guardian of_____ understand the nature of the proposed procedure(s), attendant risks involved, and expected results, as described above, and hereby request such procedure(s) be performed.

_____   _____
(Signature of Witness, excluding members of operating team)   (Signature of Sponsor/Legal Guardian)   (Date & Time)

PATIENT'S IDENTIFICATION *(For typed or written entries give: Name—last, first, middle; grade; date; hospital or medical facility)*	REGISTER NO.	WARD NO.

STANDARD FORM 522
January 1973 (Rev.)
General Services Administration &
Interagency Comm. on Medical Records
FPMR 101–11.809–3
522–107

U. S. GOVERNMENT PRINTING OFFICE : 1976 O - 211-869

FIGURE 11–1

interventions for the purpose of improving a patient's condition and illustrates how the document enables the person to enter into the decision making well informed. Informed consent, then, becomes a vehicle for protecting a patient's dignity in the health care environment, the fundamental belief being that such consent should foster and engender trust between the health professional and the person receiving the services.

What strengths and weaknesses do you see in using the informed consent document in Figure 11–1 to foster the ideal of engendering trust?

_____

_____

_____

_____

To help you better understand how informed consent became so central to decision making, the following discussion briefly describes the legal and ethical principles that provide the basis for informed consent.

LEGAL AND ETHICAL PRINCIPLES SUPPORTING INFORMED CONSENT

Legal Principles

Among the most important legal concepts that have given rise to our thinking about informed consent are battery, disclosure, and the fiduciary relationship. The common law right of self-determination and constitutional right to privacy also are instrumental in our thinking. You will consider self-determination for its ethical implications in the next discussion in this chapter, Ethical Principles.

Battery, based on common law in the United States and other Western countries, is the act of offensive touching done without the consent of the person being touched, however benign the motive or effects of the touching.[1]

Disclosure guarantees the legal right of a person to be informed of what will happen to him or her. Several landmark legal cases have set precedents for current thinking on the importance of disclosure.

One of the earliest U.S. cases related to disclosure is *Schloendorff v. Society of New York Hospital*. It emphasized the relationship of disclosure to autonomy. This 1914 ruling stated that every human being of adult years and sound mind has a right to determine what shall be done with his or her body. A surgeon who performs an operation without the patient's consent is liable.[2] Some have criticized this case on the basis that the surgeon at that time had no guidance on what to disclose.

In the 1918 *Hunter v. Burroughs* case the courts ruled that a physician has a duty to warn a patient of dangers associated with prescribed remedies.

Both rulings were early attempts by the courts to bring the patient's opinion into the decision regarding what would happen to his or her own body.[3]

Several court cases have focused on determination of what the standards for disclosure should be. Some suggestions have been that the professional set the standard, i.e., that the standard be determined as "what a reasonable physician" would disclose. In contrast, *Canterbury v. Spense (1972)* shifted the standard from the health professional to what a "reasonable patient" would want to know.

A third related legal concept is the idea of a *fiduciary relationship*. In such a relationship a person in whom another person has placed a special trust or confidence is required to watch out for the best interests of the other party. Most health professional and patient (or client) relationships are considered to be this type. The physician-patient relationship in the United States was ruled a fiduciary relationship in a 1974 case, *Miller v. Kennedy*, on the basis of the "ignorance and helplessness of the patient regarding his own physical condition."[4] This is, of course, an outdated understanding of the patient as "ignorant and helpless," but that does not negate the basic idea of the need for faithfulness on the part of all health professionals.

The case that gave to posterity the term "informed consent" is *Salgo v. Leland Stanford Board of Trustees* (1957). It stated that the physician violates his or her legal duty by withholding information necessary for a patient to make a rational decision regarding care. In addition the physician must disclose "all the facts which materially affect the patient's rights and interests and the risks, hazard and danger, if any."[5] With this ruling the U.S. courts firmly wedded the notion of self-determination with that of a positive obligation to warn of known damages or harm.

Ethical Principles

Beauchamp and Faden note that "As the idea of informed consent evolved, discussion of appropriate (ethical) guidelines moved increasingly from a narrow focus on the physician's or researcher's obligation to disclose information to the quality of a patient's or subject's understanding of information and right to authorize or refuse biomedical intervention."[6] The governing ethical principle in informed consent is the *right to self-determination or autonomy*. It also is reflected in a legal right today. For a review of rights and this right in particular, see Chapter 3.

When you consider moral rights as a patient's claim on you, what is the claim on you as a health professional when the situation is one requiring informed consent?

_____

_____

_____

You are correct if you answered something like "a claim on me to provide a communication process that allows the person to make an informed choice." One could go further and say, "a claim to honor all the conditions, including a communications process, that allows the person to make an informed choice."

Think about what some of those conditions would be:

_____

_____

_____

(Examples: Patient and compassionate health professional in a quiet and undisturbed setting at a time of the day when the person is most alert.) Do you think Faye met the conditions that would foster good communication between her and Jason? Yes _____ No _____. From what you know, what could she have done differently at the outset during their initial exchange?

_____

_____

_____

You begin to see that information disclosure, taken alone, is not the key. The key is that the information be useful to the person in making the best decision. This is discussed more in a later section.

Two duties, those of _beneficence_ and _nonmaleficence_ are also key ethical principles in the idea of informed consent.

To review, the principle of beneficence means _____, and nonmaleficence means _____. These two, taken together, morally require you to do everything possible to help the patient become adequately informed so that he or she can make the best possible choice. This aspect of the health professional and patient or client relationship can be thought of as a contract. A _contract_ implies that each person involved in the contract has full knowledge of the situation and willingly has "contracted." When you provide information to the patient or client, you are acknowledging an initial imbalance of information between the two of you. Because of this imbalance the patient's self-determination is compromised. Therefore you are responsible for informing the person of the conditions under which a contract will be struck. Only then can both parties enter into dialogue and agreement as equals. Failure to provide the information constitutes a type of harm: You fail to conform to the principle of nonmaleficence "do no harm."

In summary the key ethical principles in informed consent include a combination of the patient's right to self-determination and the health professional's duties of nonmaleficence and beneficence. Underlying these rights and duties is the goal of maintaining respect for the patient, an overriding principle in your professional code. Whether self-determination or autonomy is the *main* component of respect is open to debate, but it is certainly an important factor for most people. The challenge of showing respect to patients whose cultural and ethnic norms do not prize individual autonomy must be foremost in your mind as you read on, since so much of informed consent presupposes a patient's desire to be independent and in control of his or her own individual destiny. Some examples are provided in later discussions of this chapter to enrich your thinking. In other words, informed consent has become accepted as a part of our ethics of health care as well as a reasonable expectation on the part of patients.

THE PROCESS: DISCLOSURE ISSUES

Let us go on to some practical matters. Today there is broad agreement that a client or patient should gain information about the proposed procedure and have a voice in the decision. There may be, however, several challenges in implementing the procedure in a meaningful manner. Some are related to the standard and amount of disclosure and others to the person's ability to grasp the situation.

You have seen that a major legal and ethical concern that supports informed consent is that a patient be *informed*. What *disclosure standard* can be used to judge that the level of information was sufficiently clear to be understood? One suggestion has been that "customary medical language" be the standard. Others, emphasizing the likelihood that patients will misunderstand technical terms used by the health professional, suggest that the standard be determined by what a "reasonable" person would need in order to make an informed decision. Finding one standard appropriate for everyone continues to perplex many. In fact the courts have not settled on one standard either. A commonsense idea is to adopt an *individualized* standard for each patient. What are some of the practical barriers to institutionalizing this ideal?

A related challenge focuses on the appropriate *amount* of information to share. In many health care settings patients and clients are directed to sign a standardized *general consent* form when they are admitted. The wording appearing on a typical document states that a patient is consenting to routine services and treatment, the goal being the best care possible. In a teaching hospital the person is also told that in entering the hospital she or he consents to become a participant in the hospital's educational programs. Then, when certain invasive procedures are being considered, the consent is valid only when the person signs a *special consent* form (such as the one in Fig. 11–1). The amount and type of information deemed adequate and appropriate in the special consent form may vary tremendously from one institution to another. When you take a position, you should take time to familiarize yourself with your own institution's policies and documents in regard to informed consent.

In the final analysis the health professional providing the patient with pertinent information inevitably must personalize the amount as well as the type of information provided in spite of the difficulty in doing so. I think that in retrospect Faye may have to conclude that she "missed the mark" on the level and amount of information she provided to Jason. Do you agree? Yes _____ No_____. The goal is to take into consideration the background of the patient and relative advantages and disadvantages of each decision for that patient's future well-being. A 1995 study of patients at two public hospitals in an urban area showed that of 2659 predominantly indigent and minority patients presenting for acute care, 59.5% (over 1500) of patients could not read a standard informed consent document. The investigators came to the stunning conclusion that "many patients in our institutions cannot perform the basic reading tasks required to function in the health care environment."[7] This in itself is a barrier to such patients' receiving high quality care unless great attention is directed to providing a level and amount of disclosure that is consistent with patients' literacy and numeracy skills.

Anxiety and fear created by the unknown leave many with the sense that unfair advantage is being taken of them. When presenting informed consent documents, you should be found on the side of taking too much time with each patient, all the while being attentive to the patient's cues regarding his or her level of comprehension.

Voluntariness

A person speaks or acts voluntarily when no coercion compels him or her to do so against his or her own best interests and wishes. For this reason, persons judged to be in vulnerable situations in which their ability to say "no" or "this is what I want" should be treated with special regard. As you may recall, Jason told Faye, the nurse practitioner, that he felt pressured to sign the consent form. What reason did he give? _____

_____

Knowing what you do about their situation, do you think his worry was legitimate? _____ Why or why not? _____

_____

Since AIDS *and* drug abuse both are stigmatizing characteristics, it could be that Faye is not treating Jason with the autonomy he desires. It would be something for an observer to scrutinize thoroughly.[8]

Voluntariness also presupposes that as persons we have a free will to act in our own interests. Some philosophers would contest such a notion, whereas others suggest that any barriers to freedom arise from power differentials among persons (e.g., the more powerful constrains the less powerful) and other external constraints (e.g., the slave-master relationship). One of the most interesting and troubling instances testing the degree of constraint that will be tolerated in modern health care occurred in the 1980s when several women were forced to undergo cesarean sections because the judges determined that these women were being neglectful of the fetuses.

Another instance testing the limits of voluntariness as a standard of respect for a person is the psychiatric practice of involuntary commitment for mental illness. This practice long has been condoned by the medical profession and, often, by society as well. The increasing awareness of the importance of voluntariness, however, has created an environment in which such patients are able to maintain control over large parts of their treatment regimen, including whether to accept medications.

Competence Issues

Health professionals have an obligation to ascertain the level of a patient's ability to grasp the situation. The ability to grasp it is called *mental competence* or *capacitation*. The criterion for competence in the informed consent doctrine assumes that persons possess certain crucial knowledge without which they are unable to engage willfully in an act. Take, for example, the act of making a will. The person who does not know the general value of his estate or who does not have the mental capacity to recognize the existence of a rightful heir is not in a position to sign a valid will no matter what he or she may know about himself or herself, his or her family, or the world in general. These two pieces of information are so essential to the making of a will that unless one is in possession of them one cannot properly dispose of one's estate. In the same fashion a person must be knowledgeable about certain crucial aspects of his or her health and the condition creating the problem to offer truly informed consent. This formulation of competency is too narrow, however, when taken alone. It still tends to focus a clinical evaluation in terms of how much a person is told and how much he or she can repeat back to you. This surely is not all you will wish to know concerning a patient's capacity. A fundamental concern is whether or not the patient truly understands the nature of his illness and the basis for consenting or refusing intervention. Appelbaum and Grisso propose four levels of competence.

1. The first is the ability to communicate choices. Beyond that, there is the ability to maintain and communicate these choices consistently over a period of time.
2. The second, a qualitatively different level, is the ability to understand relevant information upon which the choice is based.
3. The third is the ability to appreciate the situation according to one's own values.
4. The fourth is the ability to weigh various values to arrive at a decision.[9]

Ideally a person should have all four levels of capacity. For instance, nothing we know about Jason's ability to comprehend would suggest that he is incompetent or incapacitated. At the same time, the knowledge that he "shoots up" IV drugs and that he could be suffering the neuropathy associated with some AIDS patients gives Faye some reason to check out his mental acuity.

THE SPECIAL CHALLENGE OF THE INCOMPETENT OR INCAPACITATED PERSON

Most writing and reflection on the subject urges extreme caution and diligence in discerning how far to proceed with evaluation and treatment if a patient is incapable of making a competent decision to accept treatment. In such instances *surrogate or proxy consent* is sought. There are two types of incompetent patients, those who were *never competent* and those who were *once competent*. Give some examples of patients who are never competent:

_____

_____

_____

(If you listed newborns, small children, and persons severely mentally disabled from birth, you have grasped the idea of persons who have never been competent.)

When never-competent persons become patients, a *legal guardian* is appointed. Obviously such a person also has had a guardian for other purposes, and in most instances the same person is appointed. The next of kin usually but not always is considered the most qualified to be the guardian. The goal here is to determine who can speak for the best interests of this person who has never been in a position to voice her or his informed wishes. (This is called the *best interests standard*.) In the case of persons who were once competent (e.g., those who have organic brain damage that developed in later life or adult psychoses), a guardian may also be appointed. You must then attempt to make your decision on the basis of what a person would have wanted when competent. (This is called a *substituted judgment standard*.) Sometimes a next of kin or other person makes statements that reflect what the guardian believes the patient said when he or she was competent. Often this is helpful evidence of what a now incapacitated person would want. Other signs are letters, past conversations, comments about other incapacitated people, or general lifestyle.

In recent years proxy consent for once competent persons has been further formalized by the advent of *advance directives*. The general idea is to allow each person while still competent to make his or her wishes known regarding decisions that will be made at a time when he or she becomes incapacitated, especially in illnesses that will end in death. Some types of advance directives include living wills, durable power of attorney documents, medical directive documents, and values histories. They are discussed further in Chapter 12. Because these documents vary in focus, you are encouraged to check with your place of employment and also with any state laws that may guide the legal use of such documents where you live.

In conclusion the guidepost to bear in mind is that informed consent in health care should be yet another means of facilitating communication between patient or client and health professional. The document is supposed to be tangible evidence that informed consent was, in fact, given. But health care professionals generally place too much emphasis on the "form" and too little on the "informed consent process." Patients often are asked to sign such forms with little more than a perfunctory explanation: "You have to sign this so we can do the operation." In many cases a nurse or nurse's aide is asked to have the patient sign the form when in fact the physician should be present to explain the procedure and its risks to the patient and to answer any questions. Many people have the misconception that if a patient signs the form, consent is legally binding no matter what. The form alone is only evidence that the patient signed a piece of paper. The forms are widely used and are helpful *if* they remind us of our obligations regarding informed consent. But in a busy health care setting, where patients' rights may be getting in the way of the efficient operation of the institution, there is a great risk that the consent form becomes an empty substitute for truly informed consent.

INFORMED CONSENT IN RESEARCH

To help focus your attention on this aspect of informed consent, consider an informed consent form used for research, shown in Figure 11–2.

Almost every experimental procedure within the health care setting necessitates some infringement on a person's physical or psychological independence. If the dignity of a person being subjected to an experimental pro-

RESPONSIBLE INVESTIGATOR:

TITLE OF PROTOCOL:

TITLE OF CONSENT FORM *(if different from protocol):*

I have been asked to participate in a research study that is investigating *(describe purpose of study)*. In participating in this study I agree to *(describe briefly and in lay terms procedures to which subject is consenting).*

I understand that

a) The possible risks of this procedure include *(list known risks or side effects; if none, so state)*. Alternative treatments include *(list alternative treatments and briefly describe advantages and disadvantages of each; if none, so state).*

b) The possible benefits of this study to me are *(enumerate; if none, so state).*

c) Any questions I have concerning my participation in this study will be answered by *(list names and degrees of people who will be available to answer questions).*

d) I may withdraw from the study at any time without prejudice.

e) The results of this study may be published, but my name or identity will not be revealed and my records will remain confidential unless disclosure of my identity is required by law.

f) My consent is given voluntarily without being coerced or forced.

g) In the event of physical injury resulting from the study, medical care and treatment will be available at this institution.

For eligible veterans, compensation (damages) may be payable under 38USC 351 or, in some circumstances, under the Federal Tort claims Act.

For non-eligible veterans and non-veterans, compensation would be limited to situations where negligence occurred and would be controlled by the provisions of the Federal Tort Claims Act.

For clarification of these laws, contact the District Counsel (213) 824-7379.

DATE _____   PATIENT OR RESPONSIBLE PARTY _____

PATIENT'S SOCIAL SECURITY NUMBER _____

AUDITOR/WITNESS _____

INVESTIGATOR/PHYSICIAN REPRESENTATIVE _____

FIGURE 11–2 Human Studies Consent Form.   *Figure continued on following page*

Protocol C.A.V.: A pilot study to evaluate short-course irradiation to small cell bronchogenic carcinoma with combination chemotherapy including the drugs Cytoxan, Adriamycin, and vincristine, and prophylactic brain irradiation. The drugs are to be started on Day 1 with the irradiation and repeated on Day 29 and thereafter every 21 days for 6 cycles.

You have been found to have a tumor of the lung which is best treated by drugs because of the extent of disease, metastases, involvement of the lymph glands or _____ .

Antitumor drugs (chemotherapy) have been found to be effective in slowing tumor growth, but are not curative as of now. New drugs and various combinations of new and current antitumor drugs are being tried in the hope of finding better drugs and more effective combinations. The aim of the treatment is to slow or to halt the spread of disease and permit you a longer period of relative well-being.

Radiation therapy is also a proven effective method of killing tumor cells. In this treatment plan for lung cancer, the affected lung will be irradiated for three weeks to maximize the potential reduction of your tumor. Your brain will also be treated with a modest dose of irradiation in order to ward off the spread of disease to this area. A temporary loss of hair may be expected within the field of irradiation.

You will also be given chemotherapy drugs (Cytoxan, Adriamycin, and vincristine) in combination with the irradiation. These drugs will be given to you intravenously on Day 1 and 29 of treatment and thereafter every 21 days for 6 cycles.

Antitumor drugs, such as the ones used in this plan, and radiation therapy may produce some damage to normal cells in the body, even though the treatments are designed to attack primarily the tumor cells. Care will be used to try to minimize the effect of the damage to your normal cells. The particular forms of damage include: nausea, vomiting, diarrhea, lowered white blood cell count, mouth ulcers, and loss of hair. The drug Adriamycin might make worse any cardiac problems you have. During the treatment you will be monitored carefully with blood tests, urine examination, x-ray examination, ECG, chemical tests, and other studies. Should any of these untoward effects occur, your treatment plan will be reevaluated and, if necessary, modified.

If you have any questions, these will be answered prior to starting the treatment program. You are under no obligation to join this study. You will continue to be treated if you refuse. You are free to withdraw your consent to participate in the study at any time without any prejudice to your continued medical care. The confidential nature of your case will be maintained.

I have read the information contained on this page and all my questions have been answered to my satisfaction. I consent to participate in this medical study.

_____
Patient's Signature   Date

_____
Witness (Investigator)   Date

_____
Witness   Date

FIGURE 11–2 *Continued*

cedure is to be preserved and his or her personal freedom recognized, he or she must be allowed to grant consent to the procedure. In short, persons must not be involuntarily submitted to experimental procedures. Rather they must freely and willingly give their consent to the procedure, even though there may be little personal risk involved. By granting consent the patient agrees to the means used to bring about the investigator's desired end and expresses willingness to participate in bringing about that end.

There are two types of research: One is *therapeutic research*, the research directed to an identified patient or client for whom all known interventions already have failed, and the other is *nontherapeutic research*, which is directed to finding better treatments or diagnostic procedures for future use.

Suppose a patient has a disease with no known cure and the investigator would like to enroll the patient in a study testing a new medication that may work. This is _____ _____ (answer: therapeutic research).

Regardless of the structure of the research (whether it is therapeutic or nontherapeutic), informed consent is an essential safeguard of the rights of the research subject. Following are the basic ethical and legal stipulations involved in both:

1. An investigator cannot perform a research procedure, even of no or minimal risk, without the subject's consent.
2. Consent is meaningful only if it is based on relevant information and is uncoerced.
3. Consent may be a necessary, but not sufficient, condition for the investigator to proceed. (For example, homicide is not justified in spite of a subject's consent.)[10]

The procedure by which consent is brought about is to inform the patient of the range of benefits and risks related to the procedures. The consent form must be signed by the patient, rendering him or her also a research subject.

What about people who for some reason cannot give consent for experimentation? Can consent be given on their behalf by someone who is judged to have the person's interests in mind? Because of the possibilities for abuse of such persons, considerable attention has been devoted in recent years to trying to set up reasonable guidelines for ensuring their protection. There is still much disagreement about the morally acceptable way to proceed. Most discussion has taken place within the context of research on children and mentally retarded persons as well as prisoners, students, or others who are in a compromised position or in no position to refuse. Sometimes they are referred to collectively as "vulnerable populations." At one extreme is the position that people in vulnerable populations should not be subjected to research unless it is related to their own illness (i.e., it must be therapeutic research). This implies that a parent or other guardian cannot second-guess what the person would do if given the opportunity to consent to a nontherapeutic research project.

Others argue that this position is too conservative regarding experimentation in children and mentally retarded persons. For instance, it excludes the possibility of obtaining values for various body fluids in healthy newborns. Without this information newborns with life-threatening conditions may die because there is insufficient data to judge the degree of their problem. This may be an instance in which the minimal risks involved (taking body fluids from normal newborns without their consent) are overridden by the great benefits gained by the research.

One suggestion is that in some instances "proxy consent" (i.e., consent given on behalf of someone else) is warranted. One ethicist has suggested the following question as a guide: "What should this person want to do?" It has been considered a reasonable possibility that a child or mentally retarded person should want to participate in research that would help others as long as it does not incur too great a risk to him or her.[11]

The above discussion points to the difficulty of arriving at a policy position to meet at least the basic requirements of morality for a wide range of investigators. As in most areas of ethical reflection in the health professions, the dilemmas around clinical research on patients are not easily resolved. Health professionals are challenged with continual weighing and decision making in their attempts to help maintain cherished values.

One institutional mechanism that has become a regular means of monitoring the quality of informed consent in research is the *institutional review board* (IRB). The IRB was implemented in the 1980s to help assure not only that persons consenting to research understood what they were getting into but also that the research project itself was ethical in its design and inception. In addition to informed consent considerations, the IRB of the institution must assess the necessity of the project, the type of findings that will result, and the way that the subjects will be treated during this study. It also assesses whether the study involves any inhumane treatment of individuals or groups. If you are asked to do a human subjects study as a part of your professional preparation, you probably will have to fill out the forms required by your local IRB.

Like the informed consent form itself, completing the necessary forms for the IRB does not assure that humane practices in human subject research will be followed. It does, however, at least submit the investigator to the rigors of review by a panel of concerned professionals and lay people.

SENSITIVITY TO CULTURAL AND OTHER DIFFERENCES

An ethical challenge as a health professional is to be as sensitive as possible to informed consent issues in the context of different cultures, whether it be for treatment or experimentation. The emphasis on individual autonomy and the right of the patient to receive information about his or her illness is a Western-European notion. Even within the United States and Western Europe there will be many different ethnic, cultural, and religious groups whose beliefs vary from the standard Northern European emphasis on individual autonomy and the right to information. For instance, in his book *Duty and Healing: Foundations of a Jewish Bioethic,* Benjamin Freedman argues that within Jewish medical ethics the central concern is of duty, not of what individual rights might be. From your study of ethical theory you know that an emphasis on *duties* is a sign that the _____ approach is being employed. (If you answered "deontological" you have done well in remembering this important foundational concept.) Of course, an emphasis on duty could lead to practices consistent with obtaining informed consent. It is still a matter of debate within Jewish ethics, however, whether an individual should make independent decisions or should always defer to the physicians' judgment.[12]

Ramsden tells a story of a patient with lung cancer who lived in a mid-America town but who had been born in a small rural community in South America. He and his wife continued to live according to a belief system that pervaded their culture, retaining their national customs and traditions as well as the language. This patient did not ask about the nature of his illness, and the family insisted that he not be told. After considerable effort the health professional learned that in this patient's native country it is considered inhumane to burden the person with information about the illness. Even so, Ramsden notes, one must be careful not to stereotype South Americans as a group. There are more than 1500 language groups on this continent, and numerous religious and ethnic groups.[13] The type of experience that Ramsden describes and her reflections about the variations within groups should be reminders that individual preferences do not stand outside of cultural, religious, and other values.

There is a growing body of inquiry about the customs and culture of numerous immigrant groups within the United States and Canada. Surprisingly, however, little research has been done overall on the variability of patients' wishes and values within minority subgroups. A particularly helpful study entitled Western Bioethics on the Navajo Reservation: Benefit or Harm? highlights the idea that informed consent and advanced directives may have a harmful effect on Navajo patients. The investigators learned that discussing bad news conflicts with the Navajo concept of Hózhó and is viewed as potentially harmful by these Navajo subjects. Policies complying with the Patient Self-Determination Act, intended to expose all hospitalized Navajo patients to advanced care planning, are ethically troublesome and warrant evaluation. In this culture then the helpfulness is related to Hózhó, which combines "concepts of beauty, goodness, or harmony, and everything that is positive or ideal."[14] Other studies have demonstrated that the well-intentioned principles of informed consent are not universally beneficial to patients even in our own pluralistic society.[15-18] These findings should be caveats to health professionals who feel confident that all patients must be engaged in an informed consent process.

SUMMARY

Informed consent in health care and human subjects research has become a standard part of Western health care practice and policy. Addressing the shortcomings and adopting varying approaches in different situations are challenges that must be met since informed consent is here to stay.

Schematically, the idea of informed consent has two dimensions (Fig. 11–3). The advent of advance directives and surrogate decision making is an apt reminder of your responsibility for understanding and abiding by the patient's considered wishes. Sensitivity to differences occasioned by the many variables that differentiate patients will be as great a challenge as respecting their dignity through honoring informed consent.

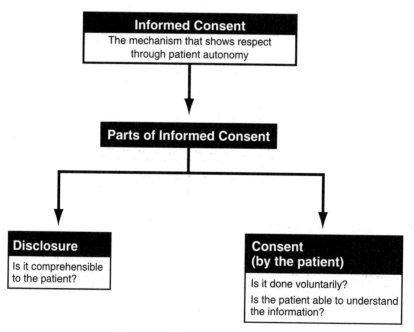

FIGURE 11-3 The two dimensions of informed consent.

Questions for Thought and Discussion

1. The wife of an Asian immigrant requested that her husband not be told that his kidney cancer was fatal. She explained that in her homeland it would be considered inappropriate to burden a patient with such unfortunate news. The American surgeon felt uncomfortable withholding this information from a patient. What should she do?

2. Describe a clinical research project that could be conducted within your health profession. Evaluate it according to the potential risks and benefits to the patients or subjects. Make an outline of what you believe ought to be included in the informed consent form so that the patient knows what is involved in the research project.

3. Suppose you are asked to serve on a national commission for the protection of human subjects. Which of the positions regarding research on children and mentally incompetent people discussed in this chapter would you adopt? State reasons for your choice.

References

1. *Black's Law Dictionary*, rev. 4th ed. 1968. St. Paul, MN: West Publishing Co., p. 193.
2. *Schloendorff v. Society of New York Hospital.* 1914. 211 N.Y. 125, 105 N.E. 92.
3. *Hunter v. Burroughs.* 1918. 123 Va 113, 96 SE. 360.
4. *Richard R. Miller, Appellant v. John A. Kennedy, Respondent.* 1974. Court of Appeals of Washington, Division One 11 Wash. App. 27222 P.2d 852.
5. *Salgo v. Leland Stanford Board of Trustees.* 1957. 154 Cal. App 2nd 560, 317 P. 2d 170, 177.
6. Beauchamp, T.L., Faden, R. 1995. Informed consent: The history of informed consent. In Reich, W. (Ed.). *Encyclopedia of Bioethics* (vol. 3, 2nd ed.). New York: Macmillan, pp. 1232–1237.
7. Williams, M., Parker, R., Barker, D., et al. 1995. Inadequate functional health literacy among patients at two public hospitals. JAMA 274(21):1677–1686.
8. Purtilo, R.B., Sonnabend, J., Purtilo, D. 1983. Confidentiality, informed consent and untoward social consequences in research on a "new killer disease" (AIDS). *Clinical Research* 31(4):464–472.

9. Appelbaum, P.S., Grisso, T. 1988. Assessing patients' capacities to consent to treatment. *New England Journal of Medicine* 319(25):1635–1638.
10. Gorowitz, S. 1988. Informed consent and patient autonomy. In Callahan, J.C. (Ed.), *Ethical Issues in Professional Life*. New York: Oxford University Press, pp. 182–188.
11. McCormick, R. 1974. Proxy consent in the experimental situation. *Perspectives in Biological Medicine* 18:2.
12. Freedman, B. 1996. *Duty and Healing: Foundations of a Jewish Bioethic*. Available only on the WorldWide Web http://www.mcgill.ca/CTRG/bfreed.
13. Ramsden, E. 1993. In the context of culture and faith. *PT Magazine* 2(4):68–69.
14. Carrese, J., Rhodes, L. 1995. Western bioethics on the Navajo reservation: Benefit or harm? *JAMA* 274(10):826–829.
15. Beyene, Y. 1992. Medical disclosure and refugees: Telling bad news to Ethiopian refugees. *Western Journal of Medicine* 157:328–332.
16. Jecker, N.S., Carrese, J.A., Pearlman, R.A. 1995. Caring for patients in cross cultural settings. *Hastings Center Report* 25:6–14.
17. Swinbanks, D. 1989. Japanese doctors keep quiet. *Nature* 339:409.
18. Blackhall, L., Murphy, S., Frank, G., et al. 1995. Ethnicity and attitudes toward patient autonomy. *JAMA* 274(10):820–825.

12

Ethical Issues in End-of-Life Care

Objectives

The student should be able to:

- Identify some basic ethical concepts that have special importance in the treatment of patients who have life-threatening illnesses.
- Describe two general aspects of humanized care that apply to decisions in end-of-life care.
- Identify three "faces" of compassion.
- Discuss how abandonment affects people with life-threatening illness.
- Describe four guidelines that can help you continue to "abide with" a patient who is dying.
- Identify some practical means by which a patient's trust can be fostered and reasonable expectations can be met by health professionals.
- List and discuss the merits of advance directives.
- Discuss several ways in which the duty of nonmaleficence is relevant in end-of-life care.
- Distinguish ordinary and extraordinary or heroic interventions and list two criteria for deciding that an intervention is extraordinary.
- List mechanisms to assist patients and professionals in discerning the proper moral limits of intervention.
- Identify three reasons medical futility is an important ethical concept and three interpretations of this term in current literature and practice.
- Describe the principle of double effect and its usefulness as an ethical tool.
- Define "palliative care" and give several examples.
- Summarize the ethical debate about clinically assisted suicide.

New Terms and Ideas You Will Encounter in This Chapter

End-of-life care
Humanized care
Compassion

Individualized care
Physical abandonment
Psychological abandonment

205

Abandonment by policy dictate
Abiding with patients
U.S. Patient Self-Determination
  Act (PSDA)
Usual and customary treatment
Ratio of burdens to benefits
Medical futility
Ordinary v. extraordinary care
Life prolonging interventions

Withdrawal of treatment
Withholding of treatment
Acts of commission
Acts of omission
Palliative care
Hospice
Principle of double effect
Clinically assisted suicide

Topics in This Chapter Introduced in Earlier Chapters

TOPIC	INTRODUCED IN	DISCUSSED IN THIS CHAPTER ON
Care	Chapter 2	Pages 207, 208, 225
Benevolence	Chapter 2	Page 209
Supererogation	Chapter 3	Page 210
Fidelity	Chapter 3	Page 211
Personal integrity	Chapter 3	Page 210
Quality of life	Chapter 2	Page 211
Informed consent	Chapter 11	Pages 213–214
Surrogate	Chapter 11	Pages 214, 217
Autonomy or self-determination	Chapter 3	Pages 214, 228
Advance directive	Chapter 11	Page 214
Living will	Chapter 11	Page 215
Durable power of attorney	Chapter 11	Page 215
Ethics committees	Chapter 1	Page 221
Ethics consultation	Chapter 1	Page 221
Six-step process of ethical decision making	Chapter 5	Page 221
Nonmaleficence	Chapter 3	Page 221

Introduction

Working with patients and their loved ones when the person has a condition that carries a medical prognosis of terminal or incurable poses several ethical challenges. How should you, the health professional, treat such persons with the dignity they deserve? The terminology encountered in the medical literature (e.g., terminal, fatal, irreversible, incurable) adds to many persons' suffering when health professionals use it in conversation with the patient and her family. At the same time, your work with these patients can be a perfect opportunity to be a positive influence. For this and other reasons I will address ethical issues that come sharply into focus when a person is going to die because of the illness.

In Chapter 2 you were introduced to the importance of care in the ethics of the health professional–patient relationship. There is no situation where this applies more than in the treatment of persons who are coming to the end of their life. Most health professionals want to convey to patients who have incurable illnesses, *"I care,"* and the examples in this chapter illustrate ways in which that message can be conveyed. It requires a clear understanding of special ethical considerations that emerge in this type of situation, rigorous application of your technical competence, and a personal adaptability to each patient. To help focus your thinking, consider the following story:

THE STORY OF ALMENA LYKES

Mrs. Almena Lykes is 42 years old and was diagnosed with amyotrophic lateral sclerosis (Lou Gehrig's disease) a year and a half ago. When she was admitted to the hospital with severe pneumonia and shortness of breath, she had some movement in her legs and could get around in the wheelchair. In spite of physical and respiratory therapy she has become weaker since being hospitalized. Tests indicate that her pneumonia probably developed because of weakness of the swallowing muscles (which allowed aspiration of mouth contents into the lungs). She is discouraged knowing that she is going to get progressively worse and die. She also believes that her husband is not willing to care for her at home any longer, a fact that the staff cannot confirm since he has not called or appeared since she was admitted.

After a two-week course she takes a decisive turn for the worse. Dr. Roubal, her physician, believes that she is not going to be able to bounce back from this pneumonia even if there is vigorous treatment with antibiotics and respiratory therapy because of rapid deterioration of the muscles of swallowing and breathing. Dr. Roubal discusses the seriousness of her prognosis, the options open to her for interventions regarding her pneumonia (medications, respiratory therapy), and predicts that she is near to the time when she will have to be on a ventilator permanently. He recommends a respirator be placed in her room for quick initiation of ventilator support should it be needed.

That was yesterday morning. Yesterday evening she requested that her treatments in physical, occupational, and respiratory therapy be discontinued and that she not be placed on a respirator, as it is only going to prolong the period of her dying. She also has requested a Do Not Resuscitate status. She repeatedly is saying to the other members of the team that she fears Dr. Roubal wants to make a vegetable out of her. He takes the news in stride, insisting she is depressed and will "come out of it."

Key questions to be addressed in this and similar stories arise within the context of basic ethical concepts introduced in previous chapters. Consider the following questions:

1. How can you show respect to persons who are dying? What, in fact, do they want that is similar or different from what other patients want from a therapeutic encounter with health professionals?
2. What mechanisms are available to honor the dignity of patients with an incurable disease?
3. How should the *duty to be faithful* to the patient be interpreted?
4. How should the *duty not to inflict injury* or harm on a person in this situation be interpreted?

You will have an opportunity to think about these questions on the pages that follow.

DEMONSTRATING CARE IN END-OF-LIFE TREATMENT

The first two questions posed above are easy to answer at the level of general good care. They need all the respectful consideration from you that you would give to any patient. They need to believe you are competent, since their life literally may be in your hands. In a word, they expect you to give them your best attention (for a review of this definition of care see p. 36).

Caring is a balancing act. As the very purpose of your professional role is to administer effectively to clinical need, fluffing pillows or flashing encouraging smiles does not constitute full caring in these circumstances. Although erring in the direction of being "nice but incompetent" can be a problem, today more often the criticism is expressed that health professionals working with people who have incurable medical conditions are technically competent but fail to show the personalized nurturing required for humanized care.

Drawing on a now classic, and still relevant, study in which many different types of patients were interviewed, Howard and Strauss identified eight conditions that patients thought were necessary for a humanized type of health care. According to the people interviewed, *humanized care* is care in which patients are treated as (1) inherently worthy of the health professional's concern. Furthermore, the patient must be treated as (2) a unique and (3) irreplaceable human being. Patients must be enabled as far as possible to (4) exercise control over the medical events of their lives, (5) share in decisions affecting their care, and (6) be in a reciprocal and not a patronizing relationship with the providers. Finally, the health care providers themselves must exhibit (7) empathy and (8) warmth toward patients.[1]

Think about Almena Lykes. Which of these eight factors would be relevant to her receiving good care? Jot them down here:

_____

_____

_____

The last two characteristics in the study are integral to assuring that you will provide humanized care to Mrs. Lykes. The term "compassion" is often used to indicate a warm or positive feeling toward the patient, which helps to convey sympathetic involvement with the patient's plight. Compassion is the motivating force that has prodded health professionals to consider ways to get around the bureaucratic rules that cause ethical distress. It is also a motivating force compelling them to want to "do something" to improve the quality of a patient's care. In addition to *compassion*, the health professional should provide *individualized* care tailored to the person. What works for Mrs. Lykes may seem offensive to another patient.

These two general guidelines—compassion and individualized care—are presented below for your consideration. As you read and think about them try to discern which character traits you have that would foster such care and which ones you can develop further.

Three Faces of Compassion

There are three powerful components of *compassion*[2]:

1. The character trait of *kindness* or benevolence
2. Readiness *to carry out your professional responsibilities* toward the patient
3. Willingness *to go beyond the call of duty*

In society we can observe these components in others, but we may not readily recognize them as compassion.

Compassion as Kindness

Kindness or benevolence is recognizable as a desire to treat people with gentleness and to "do good" when it is in your power to do so. Being able to do good depends first on the ability to imagine vividly how another feels, so that you become aware of the needs and wants of the other person. The word "compassion" comes from the Latin, *passio* (suffering) and *con* (with). Knowing as little as you do about Mrs. Lykes, what do you believe are some of her needs? To aid in your reflection, write them down here.

_____

_____

_____

If you compare notes with your classmates you will probably see some overlap. In Chapter 3 you were introduced to the idea of *paternalism* and the danger of assuming you know what another person needs without talking with him. But at the same time the exercise above illustrates well that it is not difficult to discover some of a patient's basic needs.

The desire to be kind is a resource in itself. You might find it expressed in something as simple as a reassuring arm across her shoulder, knowing she is discouraged, or a telephone call to assist Mrs. Lykes in making contact with a close friend or a person in religious life who often is a comfort to her.

Compassion as Willingly Doing Your Duty

A form of compassion sometimes overlooked is willingness *to carry out your duties* on behalf of the patient's best interests. As compassion compels you to do what is right, you can see how two aspects of ethical thought (character traits and duties) are brought together in an actual situation. Compassion, as a character trait in the type of person you want to be, aids you in the desire actually to *do* what you discern to be right. This helps you to keep to task, to pay attention to doing your work competently, and to not be careless about the well-being of the patient when you would rather be meeting a friend or golfing.

Compassion as Going Beyond Duty

Finally the motivating force of compassion positions you to exercise *kindnesses that go beyond duty*. As you learned in Chapter 3, acts that altruistically go beyond duty are called acts of supererogation. An example of such a person is the physician Dr. Bernard Rieux in Camus' novel *The Plague*, who chooses to stay behind to minister to those dying rather than avail himself of the obvious life-preserving action of escape![3]

Individualized Care

Howard and Strauss's criteria suggest that in addition to being shown compassion, each patient must be treated as a unique individual. You hear this said often enough, but sometimes it's not crystal clear how to be sure that you are doing so. Treating a patient who has a diagnosis of a condition from which she or he will die creates a challenge for you to be creative, keeping the patient's well-being always as a guide regarding the direction your creativity will take. In Chapter 6 you thought about your own personal integrity. Individualized care requires that the patient's integrity be the focus of your activity. Elsewhere Amy Haddad and I have discussed respectful individualized interaction with patients and their families at greater length,[4] so here I will summarize several ways you can test whether you are seeing the patient as a unique individual and attempting to tailor your care to that individual:

The health professional who is committed to providing individualized care:

- Takes enough time to communicate with the patient (and loved ones) to get some "feel" for the person's values, strongly held beliefs, habits, cultural and ethnic characteristics, and personality

- Thinks about how to address a patient or client: decides whether to use the first or last name of each new person, knowing the casual use of the first name may be harmful; is relaxed in calling patients by their first or last names as appropriate
- Shows interest in the patient or client but does not encourage a relationship that will lead to overdependence or interfere with the patient's personal relationships
- Listens carefully to what the person has to say
- Maintains a balance between providing sound health care services and fostering friendly exchanges

Often quality of life is used to discuss what is most important for the patient. Only the patient's (or if the patient is incapable of speaking, the surrogate's) interpretation of what makes life worthwhile counts, not yours or anyone elses. Sometimes concerns that are important to the patient seem insignificant to a health professional. What might you expect would weigh heavy on Mrs. Lykes' mind right now?

_____

_____

_____

In summary, individualized care calls on you to use your imagination, keeping in mind that all human beings are unique. What you can do for another person in your role as a health professional is limited only by your professional duties to be faithful to your professional role and, of course, your duty not to harm. We turn now to those two duties in the context of working with persons who have irreversible medical conditions.

THE DUTY OF FIDELITY

The duty of fidelity (e.g., faithfulness) requires you to take seriously all the ethical mandates and opportunities that define your professional role. Your faithfulness to them creates the trust so essential to the success of the health professional–patient relationship. Since working with persons who have terminal illnesses entails special challenges, your entire gamut of ethical resources will be useful. Erring in your faithfulness can lead to abandoning the patient or, paradoxically, to the overzealous application of clinical procedures. The opposite of abandonment is to stay with or abide with the patient. The opposite of overzealousness is to apply considered constraint when the impulse is to offer everything available to the patient, even those interventions that may help address a symptom but will have a deleterious effect on the patient as a person. This discussion addresses the ways you can be faithful to the patient's reasonable expectations (and fervent hopes).

Abandonment v. Abiding with the Patient

Health professionals seldom actually *physically abandon* patients who have an incurable medical condition that will lead to death. Sometimes, however, health professionals are caught in policies that prevent them from giving a patient as much or the type of treatment that the professionals believe that person needs. For instance, in the United States some managed care systems have been accused of saving money by shortchanging needed treatment for some groups.[5,6] Since managed care organizations vary widely in their practices, it is important that you check out the conditions of your practice before signing a contract so as not to be forced into what seems to be *abandonment by policy dictate*. Anywhere you live and work it is also important to be aware of constraints imposed by government payer systems and other insurers, sources of potential conflict by policy dictate. *Psychological abandonment* is the greatest danger. It has deleterious effects on the patient and sometimes leads the health professional to physical neglect of the patient in the end.

Psychological abandonment, such as that Almena Lykes probably is facing from her husband, sometimes does occur. Family members and other loved ones grow weary, afraid, or disgusted because their loved one keeps getting worse and is going to die. The only response they know is to flee the terrible truth through denial.[7] Health professionals continue to treat a patient who is dying, but they too may distance themselves psychologically. For one thing, their concepts of what health care interventions should accomplish may lead them to distance themselves, since the patient continues to get worse. Others are repulsed by the appearance, smells, and other manifestations of the patient's condition.[8] Some distancing is necessary to prepare for the pain of the loss when the patient dies, but psychological abandonment is distancing that far exceeds the use of necessary defense mechanisms.

In her story, Mrs. Lykes is convinced that her husband is about to abandon her. Of course, with your help he may be able to gain whatever he needs to continue to support her. No matter what he chooses to do, the responsibility for not abandoning her also falls on Dr. Roubal and the other health professionals working with her. They can overcome their tendency to flee (physically or psychologically) if an attitude of compassion is combined with an understanding of how much harm is inflicted by abandonment. What are the clues that Mrs. Lykes has reached a stage of her illness at which the health professionals might feel like fleeing?

_____

_____

_____

What steps can be taken to help assure this type of harm does not befall her?

_____

_____

_____

What additional information from Mrs. Lykes may be helpful or necessary to provide appropriate care for her, thereby remaining faithful to your role?

_____

_____

_____

The idea of *abiding with* a patient helps me to think about what the opposite of abandonment looks like. To "abide" means "to endure without yielding," "to bear patiently," "to remain stable."[9] Sometimes good care requires simply digging your toes in and standing firm.

Following are some general guidelines that can help you maintain an attentive position toward Mrs. Lykes that she will experience as your abidingness:

1. Recognize your own feelings of fear, disgust, repulsion. They are embarrassing, and the inclination is to pretend they do not exist. Denial will not make them disappear.
2. Encourage sessions in your workplace where everyone can share their feelings in a safe, constructive environment.
3. Make efforts to talk to patients so that you will know them better and can focus on who they are personally. In many instances the troubling feelings will become less important.
4. Practice compassion. The development of character traits requires conscious effort. Your disposition to want to abide with her out of your genuine sympathy (not pity) for her situation will help overcome your reticence.

In addition to these practical suggestions, you will need assurance that you are following the policies and good practices already in place to help show respect and honor your duty of due care. You deserve assurance that the type and number of interventions you are offering do honor her considered wishes and her body's potential for responding to them. Much thought has been given to guidelines that can help you remain faithful to persons who are dying.

Informed Consent in End-of-Life Care

In Chapter 11 you were introduced to informed consent. There are virtually no basic differences between how this mechanism is used for showing respect to patients who will recover and how it is used for patients with irreversible conditions. The only difference between the two types of patients is that a person like Mrs. Lykes, with an incurable disease, has an urgency to make her informed wishes known about the types of life-supporting and life-prolonging medical interventions she is offered.

The most important resources for health professionals are the information gained through informed consent and the necessary additional conversations with the patient herself. These are the appropriate mechanisms for Almena Lykes because she appears competent to make such decisions. Dr. Roubal says that she is refusing the ventilator because she is depressed and that she will change her mind, suggesting that she will want to be put on the respirator when her depression is alleviated. This is not a judgment he should make lightly, and everyone involved must follow up to make sure the right course of action is being taken. A visit by the liaison psychiatrist can help ascertain whether she is depressed to the point that she cannot make this important decision herself. If she is not, she has a right to personally refuse treatment, even life-saving treatment.

We will assume that Dr. Roubal was hoping she would change her mind, but she is judged to be competent. At the same time, when she no longer is able to make such decisions, the mechanism of surrogate decision making will be implemented. What is a surrogate?

If you recall that it is a legitimate substitute voice for the person, you are correct. If Mrs. Lykes were, say, to fall into a coma, this once-competent patient should continue to be represented in her clinical decisions by having a decision maker who functions as her advocate, trying to voice what she herself would want in this situation. This person may be the next of kin, or—in their absence—a friend, a court-appointed guardian, or the health professionals themselves. She may also designate whom she wants to speak for her.

Advance Directives

Advance directives were developed to assure patients their end-of-life wishes would be honored as much as possible. They become effective at the time the patient no longer is able to make her or his wishes known regarding the types and extent of medical intervention that she or he thinks appropriate. Because of their emphasis on the patient's wishes, advance directives are founded on the ethical principle that a patient has a right to
_____, or _____.

(If you responded "autonomy" or "self-determination," you are remembering well what you have learned so far. If you did not answer correctly, this is a good time to go back and review the discussion of autonomy in Chapter 3.)

There are basically two major types of advance directives, although some documents bear slightly different names or combine the two:

1. *Living wills* are designed to enable a patient to specify the types of treatment she would want to have and, more importantly, not have.
2. *Durable power of attorney* documents are designed to enable a patient to specify whom she wants to make her treatment decisions when she is no longer able to make them for herself. This document often is used by someone who does not wish his or her "next of kin" to have to make such a decision.

As you look at these two, what do you think are the major strengths of a living will?

_____

_____

What are its major flaws or weaknesses?

_____

_____

What are the major strengths of a durable power of attorney?

_____

_____

What are its major drawbacks?

_____

_____

The living will and durable power of attorney are legally binding in all states, but their wording may differ. You should familiarize yourself with those in the state where you work (and, by the way, where your loved ones live).

In January 1992 a nationally mandated *United States Patient Self-Determination Act (PSDA)* made it necessary for every patient to be asked upon admission to a health care institution whether he or she has an advance directive or wants to prepare one. For those who have one, it is placed in the patient's permanent health care record in that institution. If the person desires one but does not have one, the institution has forms for the person to fill out. Other countries do not have similar nationally mandated mechanisms such as the PSDA, although many share the task of trying to ascertain what is best for the patient in our present era where life can be prolonged almost indefinitely in some instances.

Although these forms are helpful in making an incapacitated patient's wishes known, far more important is that the patient talk to loved ones and professionals long before the moment of decision making arrives. There is no substitute for having had a long time in which to prepare one's loved ones for the challenge of having to make a life or death decision, as well as for having to make decisions that would honor the patient's understanding of the quality of life.

Honoring Proper Moral Limits of Medical Intervention: Ordinary and Extraordinary Means

The challenge is to avoid psychological abandonment while resisting the instinct to throw every available clinical intervention at Mrs. Lykes in an attempt to help her. Having introduced you to some problems that arise because health professionals stop treatment prematurely or psychologically withdraw, you now have an opportunity to consider the converse. Paradoxically it is sometimes difficult for a health professional to know when to stop treatment. In recent years the health professional's desire to "do all that is possible," coupled in some cases with the personal need not to "lose" a patient, have led to much concerned discussion about how to protect the patient from an overzealous approach.

In the treatment of critically ill persons the rule-of-thumb is the medical standard of *usual and customary treatment* for similar cases. Beyond this boundary are scores of medical last resort approaches, often experimental, that can be attempted. Where, then, should health professionals draw the line?

The ethical notion of heroic procedures or extraordinary means has been developed to guide you. From an ethical point of view, even treatments that are usual and customary or considered ordinary treatment in medical parlance and practice can be judged extraordinary or heroic. The ethical criterion for considering a treatment heroic is that it may inflict undue physical, psychological, or spiritual harm on the person.[10] For instance, suppose that a relatively new treatment is being used successfully for amyotrophic lateral sclerosis. It could add several months to Mrs. Lykes's life. It has disturbing side effects, however. Mrs. Lykes rejects it out of hand. As you learned in Chapter 11, you must honor a competent patient's wishes, and when the patient no longer is competent, the goal is to judge what she or he would have wanted. On that basis, this treatment is extraordinary ethically (i.e., when a person makes a fully informed decision to refuse further treatment, that treatment is inappropriate).

The Benefit-Burden Ratio

Why do patients refuse? In almost all instances a person has judged that treatments which may be promising from a medical point of view and which are administered routinely impose too great a burden on him or her to be worth it. This helps the health professional know how to allow the person to live the way he or she still wants to live, even under difficult circumstances. A critically ill or dying person often finds a proposed intervention extremely repugnant for personal reasons. Some may detest the idea of a treatment that will cause profound memory loss, that will require amputation or other disfigurement, that has side effects causing great discomfort, or that is extremely costly to the family. At the same time, the reasons for refusal may be the benefit of gracefully "letting go." It is easy to imagine two patients who would receive similar physiological benefit from a medical intervention but who would assign different weight to the human benefits accruing from the treatment. Mrs. Lykes might weigh the benefit of the experimental intervention or even permanent use of the ventilator quite differently than you or I because she believes she has accomplished what she hoped to in life and has a sense of being at peace with the nearness of death. The ethical distinction between ordinary and extraordinary rests on the *patient's decision, not the health professional's judgment.* Any intervention, from the most simple and routine to the most technologically advanced, can be ordinary or extraordinary, depending on its fittingness for a particular patient. This is the most important thing you must bear in mind, not the fact of how "high tech" or, in your view, invasive or expensive or experimental the intervention will be. A relatively simple, safe, routine, or inexpensive intervention could also become extraordinary.

> ## ANY TREATMENT CAN BECOME EXTRAORDINARY IF THE PATIENT DECIDES THE BURDENS OUTWEIGH THE BENEFITS.

The same test can be applied to an incompetent patient, but the surrogate bears the weight of deciding what the patient would have found an unbearable burden and what would constitute a benefit.

Suppose you are a member of the health care team who is treating Mrs. Lykes and it falls to you to talk with her about the possibility of starting experimental therapy for amyotrophic lateral sclerosis that may extend her life. It may also buy time for awhile so that she can have several more respirator-free weeks, but it has some disturbing side effects such as a high likelihood of gastrointestinal and mucosal ulceration. Imagine a conversation with her to explore her willingness to try the new medication. What are key points you want to cover to be sure she is making a correct, informed decision? Remember that your own preconceived idea about whether she should try the medication is not relevant.

1. _____

2. _____

3. _____

4. _____

5. _____

Any time you approach a patient with this type of proposal you should be prepared for the patient to refuse. We have imagined some of the burdens and benefits Mrs. Lykes might be thinking about while making her decision.

What happens when a competent patient refuses a treatment that the health professionals believe will be highly beneficial and effective? They are not required to override the patient's decision even in this difficult situation. In a later part of this chapter you will have an opportunity to think about what they *are* still required to do in regard to due care. Sometimes patients choose to withdraw from clinical care altogether and go home, an option they have a right to choose.

Medically Futile Care

Extraordinary care also applies when there is no reasonable hope that the patient will benefit from the care. In recent years the idea of *medical futility* has become a point of lively debate, refining age-old ideas of what medical and other clinical interventions actually are designed (and able) to achieve.[11]

At first glance the idea of providing medically futile care seems ridiculous. Why does it even need to be discussed? The reasons are threefold:

1. Sometimes interventions that did do some good initially are continued. Withdrawing them *appears* to be harming, even killing, the patient. The discussion of medical futility has created helpful guidelines for judging when health professionals justifiably may withdraw previously helpful interventions.
2. Futility always has meant that something would not help. But today there are so many interventions available that there is a need for a clear understanding by everyone of what "helping" and "not helping" means. The discussion of medical futility has led to a refined understanding of when an intervention may be withheld, although many questions remain.
3. In recent years there have been some legal challenges concerning how far to accede to a patient's, or surrogate's, demands in determining the degree or types of interventions. One limit health professionals have supported is that some medically useless treatments should be withheld or withdrawn, no matter how much a patient or surrogate desires them.

The debate about medical futility has evolved around the ethical **context** for discerning futility and the **standard** by which a procedure can be judged medically futile.

The ethically appropriate **context** is the good of the whole patient, not a single organ or body system. The rationale for this should be clear since some medical interventions may allow an organ, say, the heart, to survive and thrive, but the patient's condition may otherwise be completely irreversible and devastating. In today's high-technology health care environment the tendency to extend the arm of technical intervention, believing the machine will help when the health professionals cannot, is a distortion of the art of medicine.[12] From the earliest times our professional predecessors warned about this type of abuse, counseling always that the practice follow not only the science but also what we know about the effect on the patient's well-being. Elsewhere I have called the contemporary, technology-driven medical tendency to chase an organ or system at the cost of the whole patient's well-being a tendency to "spotwelding."[13] In many instances health professionals are responding to urgent requests of patients or families who also place their trust more in the machine than in the professional and who subsequently fail to see the crumbling patient who is victim to the health professionals' frantic attempts to "spotweld" together the failing organs and organ systems.

The **standard** for declaring an intervention medically futile continues to be the subject of debate.[14] The most conservative approach is to hold to the traditional standard of *physiological futility*, the judgment that an intervention will not, or no longer will, have any appreciable beneficial physiologic effect for anyone. One example would be the use of antibiotics for a viral infection. A second approach is to try to *quantify the probability* that an intervention will have an appreciable beneficial physiological effect. Proponents of this position suggest that even though there may be times when the intervention works, it so seldom does so that it should be dropped as a realistic intervention. A third position has been to try to develop either an individual or group *standard of quality of life*. In this position the benefit is framed in terms of a quality of life the patient would realize. Should, say, an intervention that would bring a patient to the point of responding to light and sound but never to the point of responding to the environment in a more purposive fashion be judged futile? The risks of determining whole categories of persons who have qualities not worth supporting with interventions should be apparent in this approach.[15]

Let us return now to the larger framework in which this discussion is placed, namely the criteria of ordinary and extraordinary care. The appropriate context for judging ordinary vs extraordinary is _____. If you answered, "the patient's well-being as a person," or something like that, you have learned well. The appropriate framework from which futility determinations should be made is _____. If you answered again, "the patient's well-being as a person," or something like that, you can see the connection between an "extraordinary" and "futile" intervention. Each must be cast to keep an emphasis on the patient's well-being.

Whether it will benefit this patient in this circumstance is the governing consideration.

> ## ANY TREATMENT IS EXTRAORDINARY IF IT OFFERS NO APPRECIABLE HOPE OF BENEFIT TO THE PATIENT.

You will be joining the ranks of the health professions at a time when this important topic undoubtedly will continue to be debated. At present, all three standards of futility are being applied in different settings. Any time such a standard is set, certain interventions will be determined not to be of any benefit, in other words, to be "futile." It should be obvious that the decision about what constitutes a benefit is crucial once a particular standard is set as policy that will affect all. For instance, a policy that is influenced by quality of life standards is more likely to impinge on individual patient's wishes regarding what makes their life worthwhile. The position of many involved in the debate is that when a treatment is determined to be futile, the health professional has the prerogative of making an independent judgment not to offer it. Informed consent no longer is needed. In other words, by its very **nature** it has become "extraordinary" for anyone. As an ethicist this counsels me to affirm the more conservative approaches that rely on physiological criteria of benefit rather than on the more subjective qualitative ones.

Mechanisms for Applying the Ordinary-Extraordinary Distinction

The ethical reasoning about ordinary and extraordinary distinctions requires a focus on the individual patient's well-being as a point of reference.

> ## ANY TREATMENT IS EXTRAORDINARY IF THE BURDENS OUTWEIGH THE BENEFITS
> ## OR
> ## IT OFFERS NO APPRECIABLE HOPE OF BENEFIT FOR THE PATIENT.

There are several helpful mechanisms for approaching the difficult question of ascertaining when enough is enough. The goal of such deliberations has been to provide a more humane approach to patients who are critically ill. The concern has gone so far as to lead to attempts at policy statements regarding the indications that certain treatments no longer are required. The health professions team, headed by the physician(s), is the appropriate body to make the clinical judgment about medical status. As we have been discussing, the questions that arise are not solely medical status questions, but a policy about medical status determinations can be a useful tool. Today, such policies are likely to include language of medical futility.

A mechanism to guide health professionals, patients, and their families in end-of-life care decisions is the ethics committee or ethics consultation group introduced in Chapter 1. This is a reminder that the ethical problem is brought to the committee either by the health professionals who are trying to make the right ethical decision or by the patient and his or her family. The committee itself does not dictate the course of action that the health professionals and patient should take. Its role is to make recommendations only, based on the ethical principles you have been using throughout the reading of this book and on the particularities of the case. The ethics committee and ethics consultants provide a group opportunity for everyone to go through the six-step process of ethical decision making introduced in Chapter 5. This is a good time for you to review that process, step by step:

1. _____
2. _____
3. _____
4. _____
5. _____
6. _____

There is one important difference between what you (as a present or future health professional) must do and what an ethics committee or ethics consultant does. You are in a position to carry out, or at least be on the team that carries out, the action arrived at in step 5. The committee or consultant stops with step 4 because the health professional and patient (plus family) are the appropriate persons to decide on the final course of action.

Institutional mechanisms are needed to support you in honoring your duty of faithfulness to the reasonable expectations and right of patients to have you as an attentive abider. Any policy or administrative practice that does not meet this requirement should be changed so that your best intentions to be faithful to the ethics of your professional role can be realized.

THE DUTY NOT TO HARM

Your general duty of fidelity includes the stringent first duty of health care, namely, not to harm patients. Do you remember the more philosophical term for this duty? _____. If you wrote "nonmaleficence," you are right! The deliberate and diligent efforts of many before you to put in place procedures to assist you in providing "humanized" health care is one indicator that your duty not to harm has been taken seriously by health professionals and society. The effort by many, too, to make important distinctions to guide your decision making (e.g., ordinary vs extraordinary) is another such indicator. This discussion takes you into some modern practices that more specifically express the health professions' current judgments about the morally justifiable way to treat patients who have illnesses that will lead to their death. The first two parts describe withholding or withdrawing treatment and palliative care. The last part gives you a bird's eye view of ethical themes in the current debate surrounding assisted suicide and euthanasia.

Withdrawing and Withholding Life Supports

I will use the term "life supports" as it commonly is used in the medical, policy, and legal literature, namely, to mean medical technologies that prolong life in the terminally ill patient.[16] Sometimes they are called *life-prolonging interventions*.

When an illness is reversible, these same technologies may act as bridges between severe illness and health, allowing the person to return to a healthy, or more healthy, state. When an illness is not reversible, life supports sometimes act as life-sustaining bridges between severe episodes within the dying process but ultimately are the literal bridge between life and death itself. Almena Lykes is faced with being put on life support. At this point she is refusing it, and Dr. Roubal is wagering that she will change her mind and accept it. Go back and check to see what the life support is if you do not remember and write it down here.

_____

The proper moral limits of medical intervention described in the preceding discussion provide a general ethical framework for withdrawal and withholding of life supports. An intervention that the patient (or the patient's surrogate) finds much more burdensome than beneficial and from which there will be no escape may be withheld or removed ethically. An intervention that will not reverse the condition or symptom ("offers no appreciable hope of benefit") also may be withheld or withdrawn.

Is such an act by you, the health professional, an act of killing the patient? Yes _____ No _____

The answer is "no." It is a justifiable act, the end of which may be the patient's death, but it does not meet the criterion of "killing." Killing is a direct act of commission, meaning that you—the agent—intend to bring about the patient's death and actively intervene to do so. In other words, you are the direct cause of the patient's death. In withdrawing and withholding you are neither engaging in the activity with the intention of ending the patient's life nor are you the direct cause of her death. For example, in the case of Mrs. Lykes, she has a disease that will cause her death. Her death will probably come sooner without artificial, medically applied interventions to assist her breathing, heart beat, kidney function, ingestion of nutrition and hydration, or other bodily functions, but eventually the medical condition directly will kill her. She does not have a respirator to assist her in her breathing. Dr. Roubal, her physician, determines that she will die shortly without this medical intervention, but she refuses it anyway. Her death will be brought about by the death-dealing force within her. At best her death can be delayed by your intervention.[17]

A decision to withhold or withdraw a treatment should be made openly and communicated in the medical record so that all health professionals involved in the patient's care will be aware of the decision. A physician may, in consultation with the patient or patient's family, decide that a patient will not receive a certain life support, but if there is no record of the decision, the nurses, residents, or others on duty will feel obligated to initiate it in the event of a life-threatening episode.

This type of decision is psychologically difficult for health professionals. The process of withdrawing nutrition and hydration life supports is especially challenging. Although professionals may know rationally that they are not killing a patient, nevertheless it seems so when they disconnect the feeding tube. All the team support discussed in Chapter 7 needs to be brought into play to assist colleagues in these difficult moments.

Palliative Care

As we come to realize that health care includes the provision of comfort measures to people who are dying, as well as curative and restorative treatments, the notion of *palliative care* becomes integral to good patient care overall. "Palliation" means "to decrease the violence of" something, to "moderate its intensity."[18] (It is not limited to persons with incurable conditions that will lead to death, although that will be the focus of our discussion.) What are some ways in which Dr. Roubal and the other health professions team members treating Mrs. Lykes can achieve these noble results? List three here:

1. _____
2. _____
3. _____

Some objectives of palliative care include the following:

- People with advanced, potentially fatal conditions and those close to them should be able to expect and receive skillful and supportive care not focused on curing the patient.
- Health professionals must commit themselves to using their existing knowledge effectively to prevent and relieve pain and other symptoms.

- Health professionals should regain an awareness and humility about what modern medicine can and cannot do so that patients can deal with their own death realistically, not as the enemy but as a part of life.

Clear and open communication with patients is one key to meeting these objectives. For instance, the time following a physician-patient session in which it was decided to withdraw or withhold an intervention may be filled with anxiety, fear, and uncertainty for the patient and loved ones. Questions must be openly discussed if anyone expresses such a desire. Members of the health care team must do everything possible to see that the patient is given the opportunity to discuss his concerns with appropriate support people. You know that it will be a time of anxiety for you, too, so the challenge to the whole team is a big one.[19]

Providing the best care possible means that as much imagination, competence, and energy must be directed to Mrs. Lykes's palliative interventions as you would to someone's care who is not incurably ill. Pain management is a key focus for many persons in her situation.

Throughout the patient's illness a dimension of providing the best palliative care possible (and thereby maintaining trust with the patient) involves giving emotional support to people closest to the patient. Sometimes you might find yourself becoming frustrated with the patient's relatives and close friends because they are angry, confused, or feeling intense sorrow about what is happening to their loved one, and they may transfer their feelings to you. Their demands, worries, questions, and interference with treatment can be disconcerting, especially when their actions call into question your own best judgment or exacerbate your own anxieties about the patient's plight. It must be remembered that any time the patient's most intimate sources of support are alienated or harmed the patient inevitably suffers deleterious consequences too. At best such people are a great assistance to your efforts; at worst they should not be unnecessarily excluded from your support and deprived of relevant information. They have a right to be included.[20]

Sometimes people are totally alone at the end of their life. Health professionals may be moved by the patient's apparent loneliness. I will not forget a story told to me many years ago by a friend I will call Nora Sugandi:

THE STORY OF NORA SUGANDI

When Nora Sugandi was a nursing student intern, part of her day consisted of making rounds with the attending medical staff and residents. Each day for several weeks one of the patients they saw was a withered wisp of a woman who was now semicomatose in the final stage of a long bout with cancer. The old woman had no known relatives and was never visited by anyone, but she lived on and on past the time the medical staff believed she would die. The group of physicians stood at the foot of her bed each day, glanced at her in bewilderment, read her chart, said a few words to each other, and left.

Nora believed that the old woman would become tense during these discussions, and finally she mentioned it to her colleagues. They scoffed at the idea, saying she was too weak and too far gone to know what they were saying or even that they were there. Nora became increasingly troubled in the presence of this tiny lady, who was lying in what seemed to be a gigantic hospital bed. Finally, one evening when Nora was walking down the patient's corridor, for some inexplicable reason she was drawn into the patient's room. The woman looked no different than ever—very small, very alone, and very still. Nora shut the door, gathered the woman into her arms, and held her.

The type of activity this health professional engaged in cannot strictly be called treatment, but it certainly is a form of abiding with the patient. Almost anyone would recognize this expression of human caring as the type of conduct that more health professionals should learn to practice. It may seldom take the form of actually cradling someone the way that Nora did, but spontaneous gestures of affection, sympathetic understanding, or shared sorrow can bring comfort and help turn despair into hope.

A rule of thumb is that stopping intense efforts to effect a cure must signal the beginning of an even more intense effort to engage in a regimen of clinical intervention aimed at pain reduction and comfort. As one physician stated:

> Even when we decide that our advanced technologies are no longer indicated, we can still agree that certain extreme measures are indicated—extreme responsibility, extraordinary sensitivity, heroic compassion.[21]

These words are especially valuable because often at the moment that you admit the person is indeed beyond medical intervention aimed at cure, both you and the patient may momentarily feel at a loss as to how to continue to express your caring. For example, your own imagination may be thwarted by the knowledge that the patient's time is limited. This could deter you from setting attainable goals that may be of importance to the patient. Tonight is the future. Tomorrow is the future. The patient can be encouraged toward the goal of walking to the bathroom unassisted tonight or sitting up to write some business letters tomorrow. Sometimes, too, patients are hesitant to offer information about their desires because they fear the goal will seem irrelevant or even silly to someone else. For example, one young woman confided to the priest that she longed to go to the chapel for religious services but was afraid it was too much work for the nurses to get her there. Another woman who required large doses of pain-reducing medication told the medical technologist she was concerned that the "fuzziness" created by the medication would impair her judgment when her lawyer came to discuss her estate. (The technologist in this case relayed the information to the woman's physician, and the physician arranged to have the medication withheld, with the grateful consent of the patient, when the lawyer arrived).

When your own technical treatments have been discontinued (e.g., occupational therapy, speech therapy, or respiratory therapy), you can stop by the patient's room to spend a few minutes with the patient and his or her loved ones. It does not require a major rescheduling of the work day to share a few words, reassuring them that they are still remembered.

Another aspect of palliative care is to adjust your approach according to the probable time left before the patient's death. One has to be an artist of "good timing." The person who senses that the end is near often will ask to be left alone with only a few select people or—in some cases—with no one at all. To be cheerfully intrusive at such times denies a person her need to determine the use of her last moments. In contrast, to treat a person who may live for months or years with a slowly progressing illness as if she is about to die at any moment robs the person of her sense of belonging among the living. A 42-year-old woman dying of a slowly progressing leukemia went into her local hospital for her monthly blood tests. A laboratory technician who had not seen her for several months greeted her by saying, "You still around?" She told her husband later, "She was just teasing, but it made me feel funny—like maybe I was supposed to have died already or something."

Anyone who has experienced the ordeal of a loved one's prolonged dying knows that some of the most tense moments are those related to not knowing how long the person will be alive, of being afraid that one will prematurely "hang the crepe," and of not knowing how to make appropriate plans for the future. The art of palliative care includes being as sensitive as possible to the time frame he or she is living with and adjusting your approach accordingly.

One highly successful alternative being explored for patients beyond medical cure is the *hospice* approach, which originated in England.[22] For the hospice patient the entire staff and institutional structure is directed toward maintaining the patient in as comfortable, pain-free, and humane an environment as possible.[23]

Principle of Double Effect

The *principle of double effect* is a reasoning tool that can help you in situations in which you act with the intent of providing palliative care for a patient but in so doing you have the unintended effect of hastening the patient's death. The most commonly cited example of this principle is the administration of a pain reliever that has a side effect of compromising respiration. Since the patient becomes more and more tolerant of the medication, doses high enough to relieve the pain will at some point stop the patient's breathing.

The principle of double effect acknowledges that one act can embrace two effects, an intended effect and an unintended, secondary effect. The intended effect governs the morality of the act. In this case the intended effect is the patient's comfort, acting on the presumption that the quality of life must be preserved. The inescapable but unintended secondary effect is that at some point in the continuum of this care the patient will succumb to the high dosage. Another aspect is that the increase in dosage must be the minimum necessary to achieve the patient's comfort. (This is an application of the principle of "proportionality" introduced in Chapter 3.) Finally, the unintended side effect cannot ever become the intended effect. That is, death cannot become the goal of the person providing the medication, even though he or she believes that ultimately death is the best way to achieve the patient's comfort.

In summary the most important thing for you to learn about this tool is that the intent is key. The intent to relieve the patient's pain or other serious discomfort governs the morality of the act, not the unfortunate and unintended secondary consequences (i.e., the patient dies). The second most important thing to learn is that the proportion of increase in the comfort-enhancing intervention must be only the minimum required to achieve the intended effect, namely the patient's relief of suffering from pain or other symptoms. Although only the physician has authority to prescribe such medication, nurses almost always must implement the procedures. Understandably this causes distress for nurses because they can see that the patient is reaching a dose that may be lethal. Other health professionals involved in the patient's care may be concerned witnesses too.

CLINICALLY ASSISTED SUICIDE

No modern discussion of end-of-life care would be complete without a discussion of clinically assisted suicide. Although this is often called "physician-assisted suicide," I choose my words purposefully because almost all health professionals who have interactions with patients could face patients who are contemplating this course of action and ask for assistance. Some health professionals such as nurses and pharmacists would join doctors in being directly involved in the chain of events leading to a patient's suicide should this type of intervention become an accepted option in end-of-life care.[24] Many health professions organizations have issued position statements affirming their opposition to the practice on the basis that it is incompatible with professional ethics.

In 1996 the Supreme Court ruled on two cases involving physician-assisted suicide and ruled against the rationale set forth for permitting assisted suicide in these instances.[25] What many people do not understand is that although the rulings are important in setting precedents against this practice, it does not preclude individual states from passing legislation permitting clinically assisted suicide. In fact, many commentators argue that the Supreme Court rulings may increase activity at the state level for and against a trend that appears to be gaining momentum as this book goes to press.

Most ethical debate identifies *intent and consequences* as key factors, distinguishing withdrawing and withholding life-prolonging measures (see the preceding discussion) from assisted suicide and direct euthanasia.[26] In all these the patient dies following the act. As you now know from earlier discussions in this chapter, the intent is the key morally relevant distinction between withdrawing and withholding life-supports and intervention designed to end a patient's life. In the former the intent is not to cause the patient's death, rather to honor the patient's right to have certain invasive, life-prolonging interventions withheld or stopped. In assisted suicide the health professional is the direct agent of administering the death-dealing intervention such as an injection, and the patient is a "passive bystander." The most commonly discussed form of clinically assisted suicide is the health professional who provides a prescription for and information about the lethal dose of medications. In actual cases the health professional usually but not always is physically present at the suicide. The question then is how involved the health professional must be to become an agent in the patient's death.

More fundamentally, the ethical debate steps back to a discussion of whether assisted suicide or euthanasia should be permitted at all.

Proponents of clinically assisted suicide are in a minority among health professionals, although it is impossible to ascertain how strong the support is in the general population. Proponents argue that respect for a patient is determined, first and foremost, by a respect for the patient's autonomy. It must, such arguments go, include the patient's right to chose when and how death will come. They also argue that the professional promise to abide with a patient, show compassion, and be committed to providing comfort when cure is no longer possible extends to helping a patient take her or his own life. Suppose that Mrs. Lykes requests of Dr. Roubal that he help her end her life. What might her reasons be?

_____

_____

If you said things like, "she cannot imagine going on in this condition—for her, life is no longer worth living," or "she knows it is going to get worse and she can't take it," you would be identifying themes that often are used in support of this procedure.

Opponents of assisted suicide object to the idea that respect for persons is embraced fully by honoring their wishes, important as they are. Respect for persons must entail a respect for life, and the appropriate moral role of the health professional is to save life, not to take it. Choosing to become an advocate of death is a distortion of the age-old ethical mandate of the health professions to save life. Neither faithfulness nor nonmaleficence can be honored once the line between being an advocate of life and being an advocate of death has been crossed. Opponents also assert that compassion never can be expressed by being an agent to end a patient's life in order to end her or his suffering.

Concerns flowing from this ethical stance are that the trust health professionals accrue from their willingness to take the patient's life seriously when others devalue the person will be fatally compromised and that health professionals themselves may become less diligent in seeking comfort measures for a dying patient if it is permissible, instead, to assist a patient in "ending it all." There also are serious concerns that minority patients and other marginalized members of society will be encouraged to end their lives while others will be offered alternatives. Alternatives in the form of diligent end-of-life care that stops short of assisted suicide then become the mandate guiding a professional's relationship with a patient like Almena Lykes.

SUMMARY

Decisions about life and death in the health professions are among the most perplexing, from an ethical as well as a practical viewpoint. There is much we do not understand, so awesome is it to look at the death experience. You will do yourself a favor to take some time to be introspective about your feelings toward death. Just as the light and heat from the sun are useful and necessary in small doses, so it is true that health professionals must dare to look at death closely enough to gain insight into their roles as mediators between life and death, sickness and well-being. By so doing we all will better learn how the ethical tools of character traits, duties, and rights can help to build and sustain the moral foundations of the health professional–patient relationship in this challenging situation.

Questions for Thought and Discussion

1. It has been said that health professionals who become seriously ill have more difficulty than most patients in dealing with their illness. One possible reason for this is that they have greater knowledge of the significance of various signs and symptoms related to the prognosis of their disease. What other reasons can you think of?

_____

_____

_____

2. An elderly woman with metastatic breast cancer has suffered months of intractable bone pain. She is near death and has asked her physician to do whatever possible to hasten her demise. Large doses of morphine are necessary to treat her pain, and it is obvious that a little more could be a lethal dose.

   a. If the physician were to give her a higher dose and she died, would this be euthanasia?

   _____

   _____

   b. What are the conflicting duties involved in this ethical dilemma?

   _____

   _____

3. Is there a living will or durable power of attorney act in your state? What are its provisions? Its limitations? What is the legal significance of such a document, and how does that differ from its psychological and ethical significance?

   _____

   _____

4. A patient with a rare, progressive liver disease that is invariably fatal after a long and arduous period of debility has stated several times that he wishes to end his life by his own hand "when the time comes." During his most recent visit to his physician he asks the physician to write him a prescription for "an assuredly lethal dose" of the medication he has been taking. The physician writes the prescription, then tears it up and says, "I can't do that." Then he tells the patient how many tablets would be needed for "an assuredly fatal dose." Did the physician do the right thing? Describe some of the legal and ethical ramifications of this conduct by the physician.

   _____

   _____

   _____

5. Today there is much discussion about the right to end one's own life (commit suicide). Do you think there is such a right? Defend your position, drawing on duties, rights, and character traits discussed in this book.

   _____

   _____

References

1. Howard, J., Strauss, A. (Eds.). 1975. *Humanizing Health Care*. New York: Wiley Interscience.
2. Dougherty, C., Purtilo, R. 1995. The duty of compassion in an era of health care reform. *Cambridge Quarterly* 4:426–433.
3. Camus, A. 1948. *The Plague*. (translation by Stuart Gilbert. 1974). New York: Alfred A. Knopf.
4. Purtilo, R., Haddad, A. 1996. Respectful interaction when the patient is dying. *Health Professional and Patient Interaction* (5th ed.). Philadelphia: WB Saunders, pp. 347–374.
5. Emanuel, E.J., Dubler, N.N. 1995. Preserving the physician-patient relationship in an era of managed care. *JAMA* 273:323–329.
6. Furrow, B. 1995. Managed care and the evolution of quality. *Trends in Health Care, Law and Ethics* 10(1–2):37–44.
7. Zaner, R. 1993. *Troubled Voices: Stories of Ethics and Illness*. Cleveland, OH: Pilgrim Press.
8. Toombs, K. 1997. Review essay: Taking the body seriously. *Hastings Center Report* 27(5):39–43.
9. Webster's New Collegiate Dictionary. 1974. Springfield, MA: G & C Merriman Company, p. 2.
10. Kelly, D.F. 1991. *Critical Care Ethics: Treatment Decisions in American Hospitals*. Kansas City, MO: Sheed and Ward, pp. 6–8.
11. Callahan, D. 1991. Medical futility, medical necessity: The problem-without-a-name. *Hastings Center Report* 21(4):30–35.
12. Miles, S. 1995. Informed demand for 'non-beneficial' medical treatment. In Arras, J., Steinbock, B. (Eds.). *Ethical Issues in Modern Medicine* (4th ed.). Mountainview, CA: Mayfield Publishing Co., pp. 277–280.
13. Purtilo, R., Donohue, W. 1992. Resources for medical decision making in situations of high uncertainty. *Nebraska Medical Journal* 70(10):277–280.
14. Jecker, N., Pearlman, L. 1992. Medical futility: Who decides? *Archives of Internal Medicine* 152:1140–1144.
15. Loewy, E., Carlson, T. 1993. Futility and its wider implications. *Archives of Internal Medicine* 153:429–431.
16. Daniels, N., Sabin J.E. 1997. Limits to health care: Fair procedures, democratic deliberation and the legitimacy problem for insurers. *Philosophy Public Affairs* 26:303–350.
17. Randall, F., Downe, R. 1996. *Palliative Care Ethics: A Good Companion*. Oxford, England: Oxford University Press, pp. 40–59.
18. Webster's New Collegiate Dictionary. 1974. *Op. cit.* p. 825.
19. Field, M.J., Cassel, C.K. (Eds.). 1997. *Approaching Death: Improving Care at the End of Life*. Washington, DC: National Academy Press.
20. Hanson, L., Danis, O., Garrett, O. 1997. What's wrong with end-of-life care? Opinions of bereaved family members. *Journal of the American Geriatric Society* 45(11):1339–1344.
21. Cassem, N. 1978. Treatment decisions in irreversible illness. In Cassem, N., Hackett, T. (Eds.). *Massachusetts General Hospital Handbook of General Hospital Psychiatry*. St. Louis: C.V. Mosby, pp. 573–574.

22. Beresford, J. 1989. *History of The National Hospice Organization*. Arlington, VA.
23. Woods, E. 1997. Quality of life: Physical therapy in hospice. *P.T. Magazine* 6(1):38–45.
24. Anon. 1997. Case study: In the care of a nurse. *Hastings Center Report* 27(5):23.
25. *Quill v Vacco*, 80 F3d 716 (2nd Cir., 1996) and *Compassion in Dying v State of Washington*, 79 F.3d 790 (9th Cir. 1996) (en banc).
26. Brody, B. 1996. Withdrawal of treatment versus killing of patients. In Beauchamp, T. (Ed.). *Intending death: The ethics of assisted suicide and euthanasia*. Upper Saddle River, NJ: Prentice Hall, pp. 90–104.

13

Special Challenges: "Difficult" Patients and Patients in Suicidal Crisis

Objectives

The student should be able to:

- Identify some situations in which the health professionals' ideal of compassion is challenged by the personal traits of a patient.
- Discuss the ways in which labels such as "gomer," "gork," or "crock" devalue patients.
- Identify four social factors that lead health professionals to see patients as "difficult."
- List and evaluate six guidelines that can help a health professional to respond more constructively to a difficult patient.
- Identify explanations that have been offered for why a person would commit suicide.
- Discuss several rules of thumb to follow when responding ethically to a person who is in suicidal crisis.

New Terms and Ideas You Will Encounter in This Chapter

"Difficult" patients
Gomer
Gork
Crock
Hypochondria
Malingerer
Secondary gain from illness

Noncompliance
Labeling
Suicidal crisis
Suicide
    Psychological interpretations
    Religious interpretations

Topics in This Chapter Introduced in Earlier Chapters

TOPIC	INTRODUCED IN	DISCUSSED IN THIS CHAPTER ON
Compassion	Chapter 12	Pages 234, 245
Respect for persons	Chapter 3	Pages 234, 239
Responsibilities to self	Chapter 7	Page 240

Introduction

In this chapter attention is shifted to patients who present special challenges. One group is *"difficult"* patients. With them, your challenge is to develop character traits that will prepare you for encounters with persons you intensely dislike or deeply do not understand. The second group is patients who are in "suicidal crisis." There may be additional groups, but these two will give you plenty to consider.

WHAT IS A "DIFFICULT" PATIENT?

As you learned in Chapter 12, an exemplary attitude for you as a professional is to feel compassion equally for all. This may be an unrealistic ideal, but it is important to work toward it. There are patients, however, who will wear your patience thin. This is not a new problem for health professionals, who, all things being equal, want to act ethically from the most virtuous motives all of the time! The persistence of this challenge and the health professionals' desire to squelch the behavior and attitudes of patients they do not like are reflected in this sign at the entrance of Philadelphia General Hospital:

> *Patients may not swear, curse, get drunk, or behave rudely or indecently on pain of expulsion after the first admonition.*

The year of this posting was 1790!

In this discussion we deal with the ethical problems you encounter when caring for such patients. These patients raise questions about respect for people, compassion, and even justice. Before we begin, think about some situations in which you might fall short of your ideal of professional care.

_____

_____

_____

To help focus your thinking, consider the following story:

THE STORY OF HARRY UNDERHILL AND JESSE SAMPSON

When Harry Underhill was admitted again to the Veterans' Hospital, no one was surprised. He was well known to the staff in the emergency room and to most of the ward personnel who had been there for any length of time, and none of them were glad to see him. Harry lived in a furnished room in the skid row section of town, where his veteran's pension was enough to cover his rent plus enough alcohol to keep him drunk almost all the time. Occasionally he would spend money on food but never if it meant going without booze.

This time he was admitted with impending delirium tremens (DTs), a life-threatening condition resulting from alcohol withdrawal. Often such admissions would occur toward the end of the month when his money ran out and scavenging could not get him enough money to keep him drinking. (Other times he was admitted for pneumonia contracted after spending a winter night unconscious in the gutter, or bleeding from esophageal varices, or for trauma from falling on the street or being beaten up by thugs.)

Jesse Sampson, a young chaplain who recently had begun working at the Veterans' Hospital, began visiting Harry after his acute withdrawal symptoms had subsided. Harry had some degree of brain damage from his chronic alcohol abuse but was garrulous and enjoyed "shooting the breeze" with this young man who came to see him every day. Chaplain Sampson was different from the doctors and nurses at the hospital, who spent as little time as possible with Harry. The chaplain would sit down in a chair next to the bed as if he were not in a hurry to be somewhere else. "That chaplain is the only person I know who doesn't act like he is double parked!" Harry once commented to a student nurse. Jesse would ask Harry questions about himself and his life as if he really cared about the answers. Harry told Jesse that booze was his only real friend, that his life was lonely but seemed warmer and more convivial when he was drunk. He had no family. His friends were the other people on skid row. He had no ambitions. Life was hard and pretty senseless, and he just wanted to get through it as easily as he could. He appreciated being brought to the hospital when he was in really bad shape. There it was warm, and he got decent food, but most of the people treated him with thinly veiled disgust. This often made him angry. "I'm a gomer, you know. They hate my kind, but they can't come right out and say so, so they try to ignore me. They wish I would die, and sometime I will. Would serve 'em right. But they won't care—they'll just keep on goin' about their prissy and proud ways. They think they are so good-hearted, but they don't know what it's like to live on the street, to be alone with the bottle night after night. It's my life, and I got a right to do what I want. I served my time in the war, and I got a right to be in this hospital—to come in here and get dried out and get a little food. I'm an old man. I got a right."

Jesse knew the physicians, nurses, and other team members considered him naive and foolish to be spending so much time with a person whom they considered a worthless derelict—a gomer. He harbored no illusions that he could convince Harry to stop drinking. Jesse had seen his father struggle with alcoholism and knew the awful power of that addiction, knew the strong desire for life that was necessary for an alcoholic to go straight. Harry had no such desire for life. He tolerated life, demanded his share of respect from the hospital staff, and became angry when he didn't get it. But he knew the booze would kill him sooner or later, and he didn't much care.

How would you describe Harry's behavior? Acceptable _____ Unacceptable _____ Tolerable _____ Understandable _____ Disgusting _____ Why?

_____

_____

_____

Can you identify several reasons why the other health professionals might not have wanted to spend time with Harry even if their schedules would allow it?

_____

_____

_____

The Gomer, the Gork, and the Crock

Harry could be difficult to like. But that is true of many types of patients. Some derogatory words commonly used to refer to such patients are "gomer," "gork," and "crock," each describing a type of person that health professionals find it difficult to like.

A *gomer* (get out of my emergency room) typically is a dirty, debilitated person. Harry Underhill is an example. The gomer often suffers from addiction to any of various substances. A derelict or down-and-outer, the gomer subsists on public funds. He has an extensive history of emergency room visits and admissions to the hospital. He has a real organic disease, which usually is related to poor personal hygiene, inadequate nutrition, and self-destructive habits such as alcohol or drug abuse and smoking.[1]

A *gork* may start out as a gomer but is a much sicker person. A gork is a patient who is moribund or unresponsive, generally having suffered irreversible brain damage of one sort or another. He or she may also be referred to as a "vegetable."

A *crock* can be described as someone who has many complaints for which no organic basis can be found. Such people often are suspected of being hypochondriacs or malingerers. (A *hypochondriac* is a person who genuinely believes that he or she has organic disease but whose symptoms can be traced to neurotic personality problems. A *malingerer*, on the other hand, is a person who intentionally deceives the health professional for *secondary gain from illness*, such as disability payments or time off work.)

Even the occasional use of these terms is inexcusable. Their currency points out, however, that certain general categories of patients are disliked or, at least, considered undesirable. If you examine some of the traits shared by these patients more closely and include in your examination the type of interaction they usually have with the health care system, you can gain a better understanding of social factors that lead to the negative judgments health professionals often harbor.

Social Factors Engendering Negative Attitudes

Low Social Class

Most health professionals come from middle-class backgrounds. This is especially true of physicians, but it is also relevant to other health professionals. Gomers such as Harry Underhill show us a side of life that is unpleasant and, for many, unfamiliar. Their very existence challenges the materialistic and other values of the middle class and is therefore psychologically threatening. Why doesn't he get a job? you might ask. Or, Doesn't he care what people think about him? As one physician has pointed out, "Even when the physician has genuine concern for the economically disadvantaged, he may, because of his own background [and value system], unwittingly regard the extremely poor as "different," with a flavor of "inferiority" included in the difference."[2]

Physical Conditions Engendering Disgust or Fear

Certain aspects of physical illness are abhorrent to many people. Bodily filth or infestation is only one example or instance. An old woman with a maggot-infested ulcer on her leg is likely to be shunned. This category also includes chronic disfiguring or disabling diseases.[3] An amputee, a patient with a grossly disfiguring tumor, and a burn patient missing his ears or nose confront us with the reality of the fragility of the human body. We do not like to be reminded that our existence depends on flesh and bones and that our notions of "normalcy" are narrowly defined.[4] For most people physical attractiveness is important to their sense of self-worth. We want to feel that other people like us, and our culture places much importance on physical attributes.[5] Fortunately not everyone has such a reaction. Patients who evoke compassion, especially in team members who see them over a period of time, receive exceptionally sensitive care. And so, the problems listed above are not universal. You have an opportunity not to perpetuate unethical conduct and attitudes in such situations.

Uncooperativeness

Patients consciously or unconsciously may challenge traditional assumptions you bring to your work place. For example, patients who engage in self-destructive behavior are frustrating to health professionals because their behavior suggests that they implicitly reject the advice and therefore the precepts of health and well-being. They do things that negate a health professional's help. A health professional cannot feel the gratification of curing people whose behavior makes them sick again. Suppose Harry Underhill's life were saved by a liver transplant. A common consensus is that this new "lease on life" *should* be a claim on him to try to avoid destroying his health through further drinking.[6] Health professionals who watched him on a path of self-destruction through continued alcohol consumption would have an extremely difficult time not being frustrated and angry at him, no matter the cause of Harry's lapses.

In response to frustrations a large body of health professions' literature addressing the problem of noncompliance has appeared in recent years. *Noncompliance* means that the patient, for one reason or another, does not cooperate with the health professional's program of treatment. Often this is not in the patient's best interests. As you think about it, however, what are some legitimate reasons people might have *not* to cooperate with health professionals' plans?

Feeling useful is one of the important satisfactions of our work in the health professions. The uncooperative patient denies those caring for him or her the chance to feel that satisfaction. Understandably it is frustrating for many professionals to work hard when they are not rewarded in their efforts to improve the patient's condition. Still it is your responsibility to persevere in efforts to understand why a patient is not invested in his treatment program. If you are certain the patient has good reasons for not following the recommended regimen, you have an opportunity to rethink your own judgment on the matter before discharging the person from treatment. The worst of all responses is to continue to insist on cooperation while hostility toward the person grows.

Psychological Dysfunction

To succeed in the health professions, you must be emotionally stable, for the training is difficult and the work itself can be emotionally stressful. Patients with mental or emotional disorders are threatening to your self-image in much the same way as is the patient with a physical disability. To feel compassion or empathy for another person you must in some way identify a common humanity shared by the two of you. It is difficult to identify in this way with a psychotic, demented, or sociopathic patient. Demonstrating compassion for a neurotic, manipulative, or suicidal patient is almost as difficult. Often substance abuse is one expression of an emotional disorder. It is easy to see psychological disorders as manifestations of a weak, sinful, or deficient character and to *blame the victim* for his or her disability. Professionals trained in psychiatric methods generally have a better understanding of these types of problems and are better able to act compassionately toward such patients. When an emotional problem manifests itself as a physical complaint, health professionals trained to deal with "real" physical illness may react with impatience and contempt. Consequently many health professionals consider patients with psychosomatic disorders crocks and thereby deny the validity of their need for our help.

"Difficult" Patients: Coping Ethically

Professionals in emotionally stressful situations (working with patients you experience as difficult is emotionally stressful) must develop defense mechanisms if they are to continue working. *Labeling* patients with derogatory words such as gomer or gork or crock is a way to maintain a distance from them. It makes the difficult patients objects of grim humor and thus mitigates some of the frustration of dealing with them. It is a way of saying, This patient is just one of a *type*, and everybody has the same problem with these *types*. It is an unacceptable coping strategy ethically, however, because it strips the patient of respect and individuality. It was this lack of respect that made Harry so angry. Although health professionals would almost never call these patients a gomer to their face or in front of their family, the patients will sense the lack of respect in how they are being treated.

Jesse Sampson seemed to perceive Harry Underhill as a person worthy of his attention and respect and therefore was better able to respect and have compassion for him. Harry's life history was unfortunate and depressing, perhaps, but it was his own, and Jesse honored that. Harry had a philosophy to live by and had feelings about the way he was treated by other people.

What enabled Jesse to avoid the pitfalls of the depersonalized type of distancing that results from labeling? Perhaps one reason that Jesse was able to befriend Harry is that a chaplain's role is, in some ways, to become a friend. The chaplain ministers to the person; he or she is not expected to clean up the patient, draw blood, or administer treatments. A chaplain does not have to deal with certain aspects of the patient's uncooperative or noncompliant behavior that are most apparent during treatment or attempts to maintain hygiene. The chaplain does have an emotional investment in helping to improve the patient's overall well-being. It may be easier for a chaplain to keep sight of the "big picture" than it is for those health professionals who see the value of their work only in the "successful" treatment of certain physical disorders. The chaplain also may have the advantage of presenting God as an accepting Being, particularly of those who are less well off. (This is not to say that all chaplains are better able to help so-called problem patients, but they do have certain advantages.)

Perhaps all professionals can maintain the level of sensitivity that the chaplain showed. How do you think that could be accomplished?

_____

_____

_____

When you look at the larger perspective of a patient's life, it usually is possible to attribute noncompliance or self-destructive behavior to psychosocial stresses, which are as much of a health problem as lung disease or liver disease. Some frustrating realities, such as poor living conditions or the isolation of old age, usually cannot be changed. You should do what is possible within your competence to help the patient and should be aware that there are some areas in which you are not able to help. Sometimes it is possible to enlist the aid of professionals such as chaplains, social workers, or psychologists, who can help in different ways. Even if such help is not available or is not effective, it is important to refrain from blaming the patient for his or her inability to live up to ideal standards of healthful and sane behavior. One possibility is to work out a kind of "matching system" among you and your colleagues so that people who are the least bothered by a certain type of person will be treating that type of person.

It is probably true that because Jesse was new at the Veterans' Hospital he had not yet developed a cynical or callous attitude toward patients like Harry. This is an important clue for all health professionals who strive to be more helpful to difficult patients. Stressful work such as this can lead to burnout, in which you no longer have the emotional reserves from which to derive sympathy and compassion. When this happens, you may react outwardly with anger toward the patients or inwardly with depression and hopelessness. As presented in Chapter 7, taking care of your emotional well-being is thus an important ethical responsibility. A part of taking care of yourself, however, may well be to remind yourself that striving to be accepting of all people is an excellent goal, one all professionals are called to.

In summary, there are six guidelines for taking better care of difficult patients:

1. Avoid the use of derogatory labels as a means of reducing your frustration or anger.
2. Remember that the caring function is as important as other interventions.
3. Do not have unrealistic expectations of your own power as a health professional.
4. Do not blame the victim.
5. Take care of your emotional well-being.
6. Try to help change the underlying social and institutional conditions or attitudes that lead to devaluing behaviors by health professionals.

THE PATIENT IN SUICIDAL CRISIS

A second type of challenge is presented by the patient who is in a crisis regarding suicide. Obviously this person deserves the same respect as anyone else and should be placed in the hands of professionals trained to respond to suicide crises. This discussion briefly highlights how any health professional can recognize the basic signs of and respond humanely to suicide crisis. Our focus here is not on the important issue of clinically assisted suicide addressed in Chapter 12. The special situation of a patient's desire to obtain the assistance of the clinician to commit suicide may arise from some of the same deep inner workings as the situation of someone who "threatens suicide." For instance, each may be a call for help in distress and puts a claim on you to respond well. Suicide crisis, however, goes beyond the person's request for help. The following story highlights some of the issues:

THE STORY OF ED YOUNGBERG

Ed Youngberg, a city council member, came to the emergency room complaining of severe abdominal pain. It was determined that he had an "acute gallbladder." Several weeks later, when the gallbladder had "cooled down," he was admitted for a cholecystectomy. When he came into the hospital, he was nervous about the surgery but nevertheless seemed in high spirits. Since the surgery he has had great difficulty keeping down his food and therefore has had to remain hospitalized longer than usual.

Dawn Beck is one of many health professionals with whom he has daily contact. She often lingers to talk with Ed, whom she finds to be intellectually stimulating and a delightful person.

One morning when she goes into his room, he is reading a book about the life of Ernest Hemingway. Dawn asks if the book is worth reading. Ed answers, "Well, for me it is. The old man committed suicide, you know." Then he adds, "I might commit suicide myself one day."

Dawn is taken aback, but she says, "I guess a lot of people consider it as an option at some point in their life, don't they? But you . . . ?"

Ed responds, "I've done a lot of thinking about it and have decided it's the only way if. . . ." He lays the open book across his chest and looks earnestly at her, "I've never told anyone in this town, but my mother died of Huntington's chorea. It was terrible. Terrible. We watched her disintegrate before our eyes. I decided that if I ever showed signs of the disease I'd take the matter into my own hands and call it quits before it did me in the way it did her. I don't talk to fellow council members about this, and I don't know why I'm telling you now. Guess it would be too upsetting to them." Suddenly he looks embarrassed. He laughs and adds, "Hey, don't look so horrified! I'm thirty-eight, healthy, and I *promise* not to spill blood all over."

About six months later, Dawn is walking down the hospital corridor and is surprised to see Ed Youngberg about to be admitted to a hospital room. Later that day she stops in to greet him. "What are you doing here? You decided to have another gallbladder removed?"

She notices then that Ed's face looks drawn. He smiles wanly and replies, "No, no, I'm just in for tests." There is a long silence in which the understanding of what he is saying grows in Dawn's awareness. Ed continues, "I've been dropping things. First I started stumbling, almost fell down several times, and pretended not to notice. Over the next few weeks a number of things happened. During one of the council meetings I dropped my folder with papers all over the floor on the way to the podium. Then when I was having lunch with one of my friends the next week, I . . . ."

Ed has been leaning over to pick up his water glass from the bedside stand. He takes it, but then it falls from his hands and crashes to the floor. Their eyes meet, and there is a mutual recognition that something is really wrong. He lets his head fall back onto the pillow and says with a sigh, "Maybe, just maybe, it's time."

Just then Dr. Singer enters the room. Cheerily she says, "Welcome back, Councilor! We missed you. What do you mean 'it's time'? Time for what?"

"Time for you to get busy and see what's ailing me," he says. Dawn promises Ed she will be back another time and leaves promptly. Once in the corridor she stops, trying to decide what to do next.

You may have a feeling of dread or fear regarding what she should do. There is a tremendous amount of anxiety associated with not knowing what to say or do to help a person such as this, knowing that he is contemplating taking his own life. The usual response by health professionals has been to cleave to the duty to save life and therefore to try to prevent suicide.

"Maybe he is only testing," you might say. "Those who talk about it don't do it." But then the gnawing thought that he may not be "only" testing arises.

These reactions are not unusual. Suicide remains largely a taboo topic in an era when health professionals are more willing to discuss issues related to other types of dying. Recent discussions about clinically assisted suicide have led many reluctantly to come face to face with the possibility that some persons who express the desire to end their life do it. Perhaps the guilt, helplessness, anger, and finality that suicide imposes on those left behind create an aura of mystery too awful to want to penetrate.

Common Explanations for Suicide

Suicide and threatened suicide, besides being moral issues, are addressed extensively in the psychiatric, sociological, psychological, and religious literature. These understandings of suicide have been highly instrumental in the common understanding of suicide as a crisis to be managed by health professionals. In the next pages you will be introduced to some psychological and religious interpretations.

Suicide as an Act of Insanity

It has been postulated by some writers that a person must be *insane* to commit suicide. It is not an act that would be chosen by a person having full command of his or her mental faculties. The "irrationality" is interpreted as having either a social or psychological base. The classic works of Durkheim and Menninger have been powerful influences on modern thinking on suicide. Emile Durkheim, a sociologist, many years ago proposed that all suicides are a result of a person's *social* maladjustment. Suicide results when a person's ego has been annihilated by his or her inability to live harmoniously in society. For Durkheim, then, suicide is primarily a matter of *social disintegration*.[7] Psychoanalysts, beginning with Freud, have emphasized that suicide is a *psychological maladjustment*, a displaced desire to kill someone. That is, the individual chooses to kill herself or himself out of the desire to murder someone else. Murder is aggression turned on someone else, whereas suicide is aggression turned on oneself. Putting it in a context of revenge, suicide is "revenge turned inward."

Karl Menninger, remaining within a psychoanalytic framework but adapting the theory to his observations, concluded that suicide is (1) a wish to kill, (2) a wish to be killed, or (3) a wish to die.[8] For Freud, Menninger, and their followers, suicide is primarily an aggression phenomenon that gets out of control.

Thus suicide is interpreted by some as the ultimate act of despair, the end of the road. To commit suicide a person must feel that his or her future is devoid of hope. They maintain that usually the person attempts to communicate his feeling of hopelessness to others in an effort to gain their assurance that some hope still exists. If such affirmation is not forthcoming, the person is convinced of his or her helplessness and hopelessness and decides that suicide is the only alternative. Suicide prevention hotlines and centers take this view and try to instill a feeling of hope in the person by providing support and exploring realistic options for the person considering suicide.

Suicide As Sin

In a religious context, suicide often has been treated as an evil act. For example, in the Orthodox Jewish tradition, suicide was and is seen as a shedding of human blood. Therefore it is condemned as murder. This interpretation was arrived at by declaring that the sixth commandment of the Decalogue, Thou shalt not kill, included oneself.

Most denominations in the Christian tradition, too, have long spoken out against suicide. Thomas Aquinas delineated the reasons for categorizing suicide as sinful:

1. It is an offense against oneself, against the God-given instinct of self-preservation, and against charity toward oneself.

2. It is an act against one's community.

3. It takes control of something over which only God should have control.[9]

The Hindu religion unequivocally condemns suicide on the basis that it defies one's Karma. In Islam, too, suicide is expressly forbidden in the Koran (Qur'an) because it attempts to take the destiny of one's life from the rightful control of God. The punishment for a follower of Allah who kills himself or herself is described as follows:

> Whoever kills himself with a sharp knife will be found on the day of resurrection with it in his hand, burning into his belly in the fire of Hell where it will remain eternally. The one who kills himself continues in the condition in which he died. Whoever purposefully falls off a mountain and kills himself falls on his skull in the fire of Hell, just as a woman who dies by the knife continues to feel the pain until the trumpet blast.[10]

Within Western tradition, beginning in the Middle Ages, the conviction that suicide was an evil act led to the conclusion that people who *attempted* suicide should be punished and that the families of people whose loved ones committed suicide should be stigmatized. Laws growing out of the attitudes of this period have been removed only recently and in some countries still remain. Even today in the Catholic (and some other Christian) churches, suicide is a mortal sin. Thus the religious background of the professional may affect how she or he responds to people who contemplate suicide. It may also be influential in the patient's (and family's) responses.

Summary

Suicide largely (although not always) has been interpreted as an act to be avoided. Committing suicide has meant that one is insane, evil, or socially disgraceful.

There are moral dimensions to each of these positions. For example, those interpreting it as an insane act conclude that the person must be excused because he or she is unable to act responsibly. Morally speaking, he or she is like a child. Those interpreting the act as evil conclude that in the social realm of existence the person knowingly and willingly has breached the duty not to harm. Here the greatest harm is killing, and the object of that harm is oneself. Furthermore, harm in the form of suffering is imposed on one's loved ones who are left behind. Finally, harm is imposed on society because one has "copped out" and has set a bad example for others in the community. Those interpreting suicide as a socially disgraceful act conclude that the person does not possess the moral character traits needed to refrain from this act. Such a person may be judged to be a coward or to lack fortitude. Underlying this interpretation is some hint that the person could have developed these traits, and thus some allusion to personal responsibility is implied. Some religious groups have concluded that forgiveness is possible even after death.

RESPONDING ETHICALLY TO SUICIDAL CRISIS

Most health professionals wish to act compassionately, and all must refrain from doing harm. Therefore one rule of thumb initially is to take the person seriously, not to distance yourself or change the subject. At the very least this allows you to learn about the aspect of the patient's experience that leads him or her to choose death. In many cases, merely listening with a sympathetic ear is all that is needed for the patient to seek alternatives, knowing that he or she has your support. For instance, if Dawn had spent more time talking with Ed (or would now do so) about the trauma he experienced when his mother was dying, she might be better able to know how to respond to his recent comments.

A second rule of thumb is to understand that a person's comments *may* simply be a form of testing whether you "care."

Very often, showing you care in such a situation will include encouraging him to seek the counsel of someone who has the skills to provide professional help for this serious issue. A psychiatrist or psychologist can be invaluable. Dawn can suggest to Ed that he talk to a member of the clergy. Again that does not mean that she will wash her hands of the situation. Rather it acknowledges the immensity of the issue and what it means to Ed. Understandably she may be faced with a dilemma: Should she break confidentiality in trying to elicit help on his behalf?

Finally, a caution. The health professions' ethical position is to honor the patient's dignity by working to improve the quality of life and intervening to keep someone from taking her or his own life. Part of the motivation is our concern for the person and part for ourselves. You should be prepared for the possibility that a patient will commit suicide. This requires comforting and helping each other during difficult periods. If you have invested much energy in this patient, you will feel the loss acutely. The methods of looking out for yourself and each other in this situation are not significantly different from those used in creating a support system for meeting the many crises faced by health professionals. (Refer again to Chapter 7 for ideas.)

Much more can be said about suicide, and a better understanding of this topic is needed. You are urged to go to additional sources and discuss the issue with colleagues. In so doing you will be acting with a courage that health professionals have yet to exhibit on a large scale.

Questions for Thought and Discussion

1. What type of institutional mechanisms can health care develop to foster better relationships with difficult patients? How would they help?

_____

_____

2. Patient A has a severe infection as a result of injecting heroin with contaminated needles. Patient B has a broken leg as a result of a skiing accident.

   a. Should both these patients be held equally accountable for their medical problems?

   _____

   _____

   _____

   b. Are there differences in your view of their claims to health care? Explain.

   _____

   _____

   _____

3. Several interpretations of what the suicide act really is were described in this chapter (an insane, evil, socially disgraceful, or rational act). Which of these do you believe to be the most reliable or acceptable? Discuss your position.

   _____

   _____

   _____

4. Suppose a patient you have been treating telephones you at home late one evening and, in a despairing voice, announces that he is going to commit suicide. What steps would you take in this situation?

   _____

   _____

5. Today there is much discussion about the right to end one's own life (commit suicide). Do you think there is such a right? Defend your position, drawing on duties, rights, and character traits discussed in this book.

References

1. George, V., Dundes, A. 1980. The gomer: A figure of American hospital folk speech. *Journal of American Folklore* 91:568–581.
2. Papper, S. 1970. The undesirable patient. *Journal of Chronic Disease* 22:777.
3. Toombs, S.K. 1995. The body. In *The Meaning of Illness: A Phenomenological Account of the Different Perspectives of Physician and Patient.* Dordrecht: Kluwer Academic Publisher, pp. 51–88.

4. Gadow, S. 1989. Remembered in the body: Pain and moral uncertainty. In Kliever, L.D. (Ed.), *Dax's Case: Essays in Medical Ethics and Human Meaning*. Dallas, TX: Southern Methodist University Press, pp. 151–168.
5. Purtilo, R., Haddad, A. 1990. Loss of former self image. In *Health Professional and Patient Interaction* (5th ed.). Philadelphia: W.B. Saunders, pp. 120–123.
6. Lucey, M.R., Beresford T.P. 1997. Ethical considerations regarding orthotopic liver transplantation for alcoholic patients. *Advances in Bioethics* 3:119–129.
7. Durkheim, E. 1951. *Suicide*. New York: Macmillan, p. 282 ff.
8. Menninger, K. 1938. *Man Against Himself*. New York: Harcourt, Brace and World, p. 24 ff.
9. Aquinas, T. Of murder: Whether it is lawful to kill oneself. In *Summa Theologica: First Complete American Edition*. (1947). Vol. 2: Containing second part of the third part, QQ 1–90. New York: Benziger Brothers, pp. 1468–1470.
10. Qur'an, Sura 3:139.

Ethical Dimensions of the Social and Institutional Contexts of Health Care

14

Distributive Justice: Clinical Sources of Claims for Health Care

Objectives

The student should be able to:

- Compare "microallocation" and "macroallocation" concepts.
- Distinguish the contexts in which fairness considerations and distributive justice considerations should be employed.
- Identify the principles in ethical dilemmas related to allocation decisions.
- Describe two types of situations in the health care arena in which fairness is required.
- Discuss the general rule of thumb regarding distributive justice: Treat similar cases similarly.
- Identify and evaluate three justice-related policy approaches to the allocation of health care services.
- Define "rationing."
- List and critique five criteria for a morally acceptable approach to rationing of health care resources.

New Terms and Ideas You Will Encounter in This Chapter

Allocation of health
  care resources
Microallocation
Macroallocation
Laparotomy
Principle of fairness
Entitlement

Universal access to health care
  benefits
Justice according to need
Justice according to merit
Rationing
Random selection (lottery approach)

This Chapter Introduced in Earlier Chapters

	INTRODUCED IN	DISCUSSED IN THIS CHAPTER ON
Beneficence	Chapter 3	Pages 255, 256
Do no harm	Chapter 3	Page 256
Medical futility	Chapter 12	Page 256
Extraordinary (heroic) care	Chapter 12	Page 256
Justice	Chapter 3	Page 257
Rights	Chapter 3	Page 258
Hippocratic Oath	Chapter 1	Page 255

Introduction

As this book is being published the United States has reached the $1T (that's *trillion*) mark in terms of annual expenditures for health care; the question of whether health care is a right continues to be debated; and as the number of possible interventions increases, managed care arrangements place caps on what a patient is eligible to receive. Almost all industrial nations face questions of limited resources and escalating costs. These issues worldwide create ethical challenges involving *the allocation of health care resources*.

Some of the important issues are best addressed by examining your direct caregiving role. For example, you may be faced with a personnel shortage on your unit some day and will have to decide where to cut corners and why. You had an opportunity to consider this type of problem in Chapter 8 when Maureen was faced with four patients to treat but could only accept one patient. (As you recall, her personal dilemma was heightened by the fact that one patient, Daniela Green, also was a friend.) You may work where there are not enough instruments or personnel to fully satisfy what your best effort requires. In deciding how to operate under that extenuating circumstance you are again making allocation decisions. These are termed *microallocation* decisions.

But some of the most critical issues regarding allocation of resources removes you from the arena of direct patient care to policy, where whole groups of like-situated people are considered. For instance, one current lively policy debate surrounds liver transplantation. There is a serious shortage of available donor livers. The greatest number of patients needing transplantation for survival are those suffering from alcohol-related end-stage liver disease.[1] There have been many debates regarding the ethical responsibility to provide transplants to alcoholic patients. What do you think? Should a person whose liver has been damaged by alcohol or other substance abuse have the same chance of a transplant as someone whose liver damage was due to disease not lifestyle? What do you think? Yes _____ No _____

If yes, list any conditions you would impose on the substance abuser to try to assure that he or she would not end up in the same situation again? Conversely, if you think a person who is an alcoholic should be given exactly the same priority as anyone else with similar medical need, explain your position here._____

_____

_____

Presently in most countries where liver transplants are offered there is a waiting period for alcoholics to demonstrate that they are abstaining from alcohol, a criterion that appears to reduce the recidivism rate among those fortunate enough to be chosen for an organ.[2] Whatever the outcome, the decision about organ transplantation points out that in the allocation of health care resources conscious choices are made, and the choices do make a difference in the lives and well-being of whole groups of like-situated people.[3]

Some policy decisions require that different types of societal goods be compared. For instance, an allocation decision may be required to decide whether during this year more roads will be built, or hospice beds increased, or existing national parks maintained. These decisions are called *macroallocation* decisions.

As usual, I am presenting you with a case to assist you in your thinking about these complex practice and policy issues. The emphasis will be on microallocation decisions, although both will be addressed.

THE STORY OF MR. LACEY AND HIS RIGHT TO REMAIN IN THE ICU

One Monday morning as John Krescher, a critical care nurse, is going into the intensive care unit (ICU), he is stopped by Mr. Lacey's sister. John often has seen her and her husband there at her brother's bedside, although they have not had any lengthy discussions about Mr. Lacey. This morning she says angrily that Dr. McCally is planning to transfer her brother prematurely to the general medical unit because he is being urged to do so by the hospital utilization committee as well as the case manager for Mr. Lacey's managed care plan. She and her husband are threatening a lawsuit against the hospital unless Mr. Lacey is allowed to remain in the ICU and receive the fullest medical care there. John expresses his surprise and is about to ask her some further questions, but she rushes out of the unit, apparently on the verge of tears.

John goes over to Mr. Lacey's bedside and puts his hand on the man's shoulder. He studies Mr. Lacey's face for some sign of response, but there is none. John's mind is flooded with thoughts. Mr. Lacey is a 28-year-old, divorced postal employee with no children. "He is only a year older than I am," John thinks. Initially Mr. Lacey was admitted to the hospital complaining of severe, acute abdominal pain. After several days of tests that yielded no clues, the physicians did an exploratory laparotomy.* At that time an ischemic segment of bowel was resected. In the postoperative suite Mr. Lacey experienced respiratory arrest for reasons the doctors could not understand and was transferred to the ICU. Since that time, three weeks ago, he has been in a fluctuating level of coma and has never fully regained consciousness.

Mr. Lacey has had a stormy course characterized by multiple serious medical complications. He developed a severe systemic infection immediately after surgery, at which time it was thought he would die. He was treated with massive doses of antibiotics and appeared recovered. But the antibiotics were severely toxic to his kidneys. He is now showing signs of renal failure, which may necessitate dialysis.

Some members of the health care team have become progressively more pessimistic about Mr. Lacey's prognosis. In the ICU rounds two days ago Dr. McCally shared with the ICU nursing staff that he had had several discussions with Mr. Lacey's sister and had tried to explain to her the unlikelihood that Mr. Lacey's condition would improve. "But," Dr. McCally said, "she and her husband wish aggressive treatment as long as there is any hope of meaningful recovery or survival." Mr. Lacey had left no living will or durable power of attorney and had never expressed an opinion about long-term life support.

John goes back to the ICU desk where his colleague Janet Cumming is at the computer entering data in the patient medical records. Janet says, "Mr. Lacey's sister is so upset because Dr. McCally has been ordered to discontinue intensive care therapy in spite of the family's objections. We will be transferring him back to the regular medicine unit later today. My guess is that he will die there. Of course, we *are* 100% full, so I can see why there is a push to get him out, but he is being discharged from us before he is ready."

This story raises a number of ethical questions. A seemingly healthy younger man becomes a victim of a series of events that leave him in a coma and dependent on medical life supports for his life and sustenance. What should be done for this man who shows no improvement and seems to be getting worse? Of the many issues involved in this situation, consider the following that are related to the broad questions of allocation of health care resources:

1. Should care be continued in the ICU for people who will get worse if they are transferred out but who do not seem to be getting any better?
2. Should Mr. Lacey be continued in the ICU because the family has a right to require continued treatment of this sort?

---

*A *laparotomy* is a procedure in which a surgeon enters the abdominal cavity to discover the source of a serious problem not detectable by other means.

3. Should Mr. Lacey be transferred out because his health plan guidelines dictate that he has used up his fair share of the plan's resources, and besides, this regimen for him is based on data derived from many other people who supposedly were in circumstances similar to his?
4. Should his financial situation be a factor in whether he is kept in the ICU?

A widely recognized goal for health professionals is to do whatever is "best" or, in the language of ethics, *beneficent* for the patient. In this story the entire team has been working to make sure that Mr. Lacey is receiving the best care each is able to provide. It is what we expect of the health professional–patient relationship.

In recent years, however, the direct relationship between health professional and patient has become strained by institutional constraints. Traditional health care ethics, with its emphasis only on the private transaction between you and the patient, often has not addressed the larger institutional questions. For instance, there is nothing in the Hippocratic Oath or even in most professional codes of ethics that provides guidance for how to distribute health care resources fairly. The challenge is heightened when the allocation involves a scarce resource.

THE ONE AND THE MANY: FAIRNESS CONSIDERATIONS

Patients such as Mr. Lacey bring the troubling aspects of resource allocation keenly into focus. Although theoretically it is possible to keep Mr. Lacey alive indefinitely, the reality is that the technology required to keep him alive in the ICU is expensive. One problem is the uncertainty about whether Mr. Lacey will die if removed from the ICU, although it appears that he cannot go on for long without intensive care and dialysis. The treatment he requires is out of reach for his family financially and for anyone except the wealthiest. Therefore the benefits Mr. Lacey derives from treatment inevitably are at the expense of pooled financial resources (in the form of revenue from taxes, insurance premiums, and other common funds). Of course, Mr. Lacey has worked since he was sixteen years old, so he also has contributed to these funds over the years, with the knowledge that he himself might not need them.

There are two issues raised by Mr. Lacey's situation that require an understanding of the *principle of fairness*:

First, resources he requires may keep someone else from receiving this valued life-saving therapy in the ICU. Generally speaking, once a patient is in an ICU, he or she will not be removed for another. To intensify the problem, imagine that the ICU is full and that by keeping Mr. Lacey there for such a long time a number of other patients needing ICU care actually are prevented from receiving it. (One can imagine that Mr. Lacey himself would have died following his respiratory arrest had the ICU been full at the time.) In Chapter 4 this type of problem was introduced as an _____ _____ because your duty (in this case, to be fair) to more than one patient cannot be realized.

Schematically it looks like this:

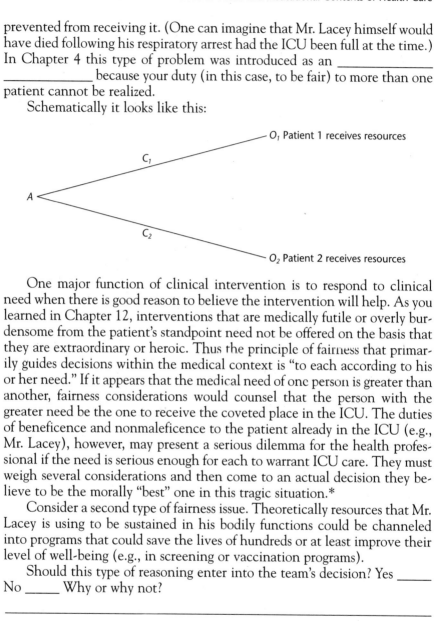

One major function of clinical intervention is to respond to clinical need when there is good reason to believe the intervention will help. As you learned in Chapter 12, interventions that are medically futile or overly burdensome from the patient's standpoint need not be offered on the basis that they are extraordinary or heroic. Thus the principle of fairness that primarily guides decisions within the medical context is "to each according to his or her need." If it appears that the medical need of one person is greater than another, fairness considerations would counsel that the person with the greater need be the one to receive the coveted place in the ICU. The duties of beneficence and nonmaleficence to the patient already in the ICU (e.g., Mr. Lacey), however, may present a serious dilemma for the health professional if the need is serious enough for each to warrant ICU care. They must weigh several considerations and then come to an actual decision they believe to be the morally "best" one in this tragic situation.*

Consider a second type of fairness issue. Theoretically resources that Mr. Lacey is using to be sustained in his bodily functions could be channeled into programs that could save the lives of hundreds or at least improve their level of well-being (e.g., in screening or vaccination programs).

Should this type of reasoning enter into the team's decision? Yes _____ No _____ Why or why not?

_____

_____

_____

_____

*The health care team's decision also would be influenced by Mr. Lacey's wishes if Mr. Lacey has left a living will or previously indicated to Dr. McCally or the family what he wished to have done.

This type of reasoning is a morally questionable guide for action at the level that decisions are being made about a particular patient by his or her health care team. In the first place, we value individual life too highly. There is no assurance that funds and other resources "saved" by removing Mr. Lacey from the ICU will be channeled into saving more lives or increasing the level of health of more people. Even if we did have that assurance, the respect for a patient's dignity as a human being should preclude the health professional's compromising a single patient's well-being for the sake of others "out there." At the same time, policies designed to handle the dilemma of scarce resources must be honored as long as all who stand to lose or gain by such a policy are treated equitably.

You will now have an opportunity to consider the same situation from the angle of similarly situated *groups* of individuals vying for a limited health care resource.

Social policy should be designed to protect the interests of everyone equitably. In the situation we are discussing, this would include Mr. Lacey, similar patients requiring ICU services, and the ongoing life of the community. The policy may be in the form of federal or other government guidelines or an institution policy. It might include directives for types of treatment that will not be covered by insurance, Medicare, or other third-party payers, or it might provide guidelines for types of patients who will not be treated because of excessive cost or unlikelihood of medical response to treatment. It is understandable that much thought has gone into determining moral guidelines to help health professionals make just decisions. The guidelines are considerations of *distributive justice*. At their gravest, such decisions entail denying treatment to some patients who need treatment. In these situations of dire scarcity, *rationing* is required.

ALLOCATIONS AMONG GROUPS: JUSTICE CONSIDERATIONS

In Chapter 3 you were introduced briefly to the idea of justice. To review: justice can be thought of as an arbiter, useful for analyzing and resolving ethical problems regarding what is rightfully due each claimant amidst their competing claims.

In society, claims are taken into account according to groups of people who are judged to be similarly situated according to need, merit, or other considerations. Mr. Lacey becomes less of a focus as an individual and more of a focus as one who belongs to a group of people requiring ICU care. In fact a general rule of justice when there are goods and burdens to be allocated is to "treat similar cases similarly." Obviously the idea of simply treating similar cases similarly presents some difficulties because you can treat whole groups of people poorly (e.g., slaves in the United States and elsewhere). The idea of justice is to show respect for people by not making ar-

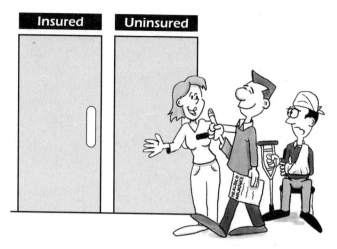

FIGURE 14–1

bitrary or capricious distinctions and by not discriminating against some groups on that basis. Justice requires that morally defensible differences among people be used to decide who gets what.

To apply justice as an ethical principle, you must be dealing with a resource that is prized but is in such short supply that not every group who wants or needs it can have it. The resource in this case may be hospital beds or hospitals, health professionals, medications or other types of treatment, or diagnostic modalities. Sometimes when these resources are available, many groups of people cannot avail themselves of them because they cannot pay for them.[4] At the time this book was being written, approximately 50 million people in the United States are uninsured or seriously underinsured for health care needs. These figures raise serious ethical questions about how our society views the cherished resource of health care and who should have priority when access to it is being granted.

Health Care As a Right

One fundamental approach to the issue is to determine whether health care is a *right* and if so to how much health care an individual or group is entitled. As you probably recall, a right is a stringent _____. The stronger the claim, the more likely a society will accept responsibility for developing policy designed to meet the claim on behalf of all its citizens. Given the present policies of health care, do you think the United States views health care as a right? _____ Does Canada? _____

The language sometimes used in discussing a rights approach is that of *entitlement*. If there is a right, everyone is entitled to a share of it according to some agreed-on criteria. Dougherty discusses four interpretations of what entitlement might involve in respect to policy:

- The utilitarian ideal of accepting health care as a right because, overall, doing so is best for the greatest number
- An egalitarian ideal based on the reality that everyone is subject equally to pain, suffering, disability, and death
- A contractual approach in which each receives whatever we as a society contract with each other to accept
- The libertarian ideal in which one is left alone to decide how and if to avail oneself of a health care option[5]

A rights-oriented approach entails policies that enable everyone to receive health care benefits. Access would have to be *universally available*. People such as Mr. Lacey and the other patients who need ICU beds should be able to have them. The societal challenge is to find money and ICU beds so that such a resource is available for those who will benefit from this type of care.

Presently there are many proposals for reform within the United States and Canadian health care systems, many of them based on the understanding that health care is a right. Most nations that have nationalized or socialized forms of health care share this view.

Health Care As Response to Basic Need

A second approach is to base allocations on *justice according to need*. Health care addresses a basic human need. Therefore everyone ought to have this need responded to. In this approach you could still think of health care as a right but only because of its power to help maintain health, prevent suffering, and alleviate the suffering that comes from an illness, injury, or the like. In other words the governing idea in the second approach is the type of need that is responsive to health care intervention. People with similar needs should be treated similarly. All things being equal, those with more need should have higher priority unless there is evidence that the expenditure of resources on this group would not yield positive results. As you can imagine, one of the greatest challenges in this type of approach is to define severity of need and likelihood of benefit among different groups, although it is the approach that most fully characterizes the ideals in traditional health care codes of ethics and oaths.

Health Care As Commodity

A third approach is to base allocations on *justice according to merit*. Health care is treated the same as any other type of product in a free market society. Many policies and practices in the United States health care arena today are based on this type of reasoning. A treatment is a commodity to be bought like a summer vacation package, or trash masher, or Barbie doll. The informed consumer decides and makes choices. One key resource that governs such an approach is money. In this approach it is not the responsibility of society to provide money (or vouchers or employee-based health insurance plans) so that people will be able to pay for health care when they wish to purchase it. Everyone buys what he or she wants and, in addition, can afford. People situated like Mr. Lacey are free to buy more time in the ICU if they are able to pay for it.

Merit As a Criterion

This approach takes more subtle forms as well. "Merit" may not mean strictly that a person is able to extract from his or her pocket the money to pay for a course of health care interventions. Sometimes the merit is judged according to the person's ability to benefit in such a way that he or she will be financially valuable to society. In other words, a group may gain priority by being viewed as a "good investment." This becomes a tricky decision to make because the justifiable emphasis on a group's being able to benefit from intervention can cross the line to become discrimination: an emphasis on people who are younger, have higher basic intelligence, or appear to be better situated to be income producers.

For example, suppose two men are brought into the emergency room following an auto accident. Both need ICU care and are expected to benefit from this care, but there is only one bed available. Mr. A., a brilliant, 26-year-old doctoral student, is on the brink of making a major breakthrough in Alzheimer's research. His ability to pay for care is limited because of his need to pay off large student loans. Mr. B., age 75, is a wealthy, world-renowned, retired concert pianist.

What "merits" does each have that might influence your thinking?

Mr. A_____

_____

Mr. B_____

_____

Because you are considering groups of people, name some characteristics of persons that you might give high priority to if you were setting policy to address these difficult decisions.

From a justice point of view, this approach is characterized best as justice according to merit. The groups with the money to buy health care, or to be a good financial return on society's investment, have the necessary qualification or "merit" required to receive it.

As you can glean from this summary of approaches, actual health care policies in the United States today are a mixture, whereas Canadian and European policies focus on rights and basic needs. It seems as if in the United

States, people are still trying to decide what type of resource health care is and on what basis people should receive it. As you read and reflect on the approaches, try to determine your own position on this weighty matter.

RATIONING-ALLOCATION AND DIRE SCARCITY

Having given careful attention to the principle of distributive justice, let us turn to the notion of rationing. *Rationing* is an intentional method of distributing a desired good when there are too many qualified claimants for a good. In other words, rationing decisions are made when there is a dire or severe shortage of the good and the conscious ("rational") goal is to distribute it fairly as far as the limited good will go *and* to decide who will (or, tragically, will not) receive a fair portion.

The decision-making procedure is based on concern for the ongoing life of the community (e.g., forgoing "inordinate costs" for one for the sake of equalized benefits to many more). Almost everyone would agree that attributing priority to the survival of the whole group is appropriate in situations of dire (but only dire) scarcity.

Criteria for a Morally Acceptable Approach to Rationing of Health Care Resources

There Must Be a Demonstrated Need That Rationing Is Necessary

Rationing means that some groups who would benefit will not receive needed services. The idea that health care responds to a basic human need requires that the burden of proof be placed on anyone declaring that it is time to ration the good.

It Must Be a Last Resort Move

It follows from the preceding that every other approach must be exhausted before persons who would benefit will be excluded from care. For example, one necessary exercise is to entertain less expensive but equally effective modes of treatment that would be offered to everyone for a given type of problem. Managed care arrangements, such as the one in which Mr. Lacey is enrolled, attempt to keep costs in check by limiting the number of treatment days and costs a patient may incur based on pooled data from many similar patients before him. Some of the people involved in his care question whether the conclusion is the right one *for him*.

A Standard of Care Must Be Established and Honored

Many groups have attempted to establish a baseline level to help assure equity for everyone. For example, the Ethical and Religious Directives for Catholic Health Care Services require that poor people be a focal point of consideration. If their needs are met, it is likely that others' needs will be too.[6] Philosopher John Rawls' proposal that an unequal distribution of basic goods in a society must be acceptable from the standpoint of the least well off.[7] Many nations have used a basic set of benefits that *everyone* must receive as a bottom-line standard, no matter how minimal.

The Process Must Be Inclusive

Representatives and advocates for all groups that will be affected should participate in the policy-making process. An interesting experiment in rationing was conducted by the state of Oregon in regard to its Medicaid recipients. A random group of taxpayers was asked to priority-rank many treatment interventions, the idea being that when the results were tabulated, the state dollars allocated annually to health services would be directed only to people needing *those* treatment interventions. When the money ran out, no more payment would be made that year. What is your reaction to this approach to rationing?

Proportionality and Reversibility Are Required

The beneficial services withheld must be proportional to the actual scarcity. Cuts or cutbacks are justifiable only as long as true and serious scarcity exists. See following criteria:

Criteria for a Morally Acceptable Approach to Rationing of Health Care Resources

1. It must be demonstrated that rationing is necessary.
2. It must be a last resort move.
3. A locus of loyalty to help assure that items 1 and 2 will be honored should be established.
4. The process itself must be inclusive.
5. Proportionality and reversibility are required.

Tragic Choices

In the awesome possibility of eliminating some people from resources altogether, a *lottery* approach, or process of *random selection,* has been suggested by some as a procedure that can help to make a decision more just when the claim is for a particular medical treatment simply not available to everyone who needs it.

In random selection a prior medical judgment of medical need and suitability has been made, and the patient's freedom to refuse possible treatment is honored. In an attempt to be as impersonal as possible in selecting who is to receive treatment among those still found eligible, casting lots has been suggested as a model. In extreme circumstances such as this the method has been upheld in the courts of the United States as a procedure that fully expresses an equal consideration of the equal right of each person to his or her life (*United States v. Holmes*).[8] It affirms that there is no way of justly determining a person's social worth to others and so removes the necessity of an arbitrary decision among those who are equally medically needy but otherwise differ.

It also has been argued by proponents of this position that those unfortunate people who are excluded from treatment may find it easier to accept because they have not been excluded on the basis of individual traits they have or do not have.

Nonetheless not everyone agrees that random selection always is the most humane way of proceeding. Rescher has defended a position in which social worth criteria are considered in addition to medical need.[9] He maintained that once patients have been selected as equal in medical regards (need, likelihood of successful response to treatment, and believed life expectancy following treatment), then three additional social factors can be used to distinguish among those still eligible. They are (1) the likelihood of future service to society, (2) the extent of past services to society, and (3) the extent to which the person has family responsibilities (to spouse, children, or parents). Rescher did not defend the use of these criteria as a system of justice generally but only in the most extreme scarcity. He takes seriously the fact that people are seldom viewed as isolated atoms but rather in the light of their contributions and relationships. The difficulty of this position is that those in a position of power are forced to make life and death treatment decisions on the basis of social differences among individuals.

SUMMARY

In conclusion, discussion of the proper moral response to Mr. Lacey's situation raises many questions regarding the most morally defensible way to proceed. Inherent in the judgment are considerations of principles of fairness and distributive justice and the appropriate criteria for a rationing approach.

What Dr. McCally and the other members of the health care team decide to do will be based on clinical and policy considerations. In the ethical dimensions of the decision, they will be faced with the issues of fairness and their duty to be faithful to the patient and to do no harm. They will need courage to act on their decision in addition to wisdom to decide well. Although questions of distributive justice are at the heart of the case, much more is at stake in the actual decision-making situation for this man, his family, and their relationship with the health professionals.

Questions for Thought and Discussion

1. Imagine that a friend of yours has AIDS and a highly experimental but potentially lifesaving medication has been found. At present the supply is too scarce for everyone who needs it to receive it. What type of decision-making procedure for deciding who should receive the drug is the most fair?

_____

_____

2. Discuss some difficulties in using the criterion of medical need as the basis for distribution of health care resources among various groups and individuals.

_____

_____

_____

_____

_____

3. (This exercise can be performed as an individual or group exercise.) You have an opportunity to argue for which services should be included and excluded in your state's health care rationing plan for Medicaid recipients. You have taken this task seriously for many reasons, but one is that the federal government has given your state the opportunity to develop a rationing plan for Medicaid recipients nationally.

   On the basis of the Oregon plan, the first step was to poll a random group of citizens to set priorities among services. Your task force has gone one step further than the Oregon plan. Oregon polled only voting citizens. You set a mechanism in place that assured input from a large contingency of Medicare recipients from across your state. (One criticism leveled at Oregon policy makers was that their pool of voters did not include a proportionate number of Oregon Medicaid recipients.)

   Now the real crunch has come because several important services that the members of the task force thought would be included are not. You will now decide among yourselves how to make the final cuts but will not mess with the list created by the first part of the process (as described above).

The task force has before it six possible services that could be included for the state's Medicaid recipients (all estimated costs are annual, and the task force has $1,136,000 to allocate):

1. Preventive dental care for children ages 2 to 6 years (includes a yearly check up, teeth cleaning). Does not include fillings, orthodontics, or other acute dental or surgical services. **Estimated cost: $276,000.**

2. Outpatient mental health services (initial evaluation and up to 12 visits) for children and adolescents (ages 4 to 19 years). Does not include medications or hospitalization. **Estimated cost: $600,000.**

3. Smoking-related asthma treatments. **Estimated cost: $496,000.**

4. Liver transplantation. **Estimated cost: $990,000.**

5. Mammograms for women under the age of 50. **Estimated cost: $490,000.**

6. Coverage for pain management for patients with chronic back pain. Includes medications, rehabilitation, pain centers. Does not include surgery, which could be covered in another surgical category that ranked higher on the list of services. **Estimated cost: $1,040,000.**

Rank order, with highest priority number 1 and lowest 6.

1._____

2._____

3._____

4._____

5._____

6._____

Jot down your rationale here.

_____

_____

_____

References

1. Kelso, L. 1994. Alcohol-related end-stage liver disease and transplantation: The debate continues. *Clinical Issues in Critical Care Nursing* 5(4):501–506.
2. Krom, R. 1994. Liver transplantation and alcohol: Who should get transplants? *Hepatology* 20(1, Pt. 2):28S–32S.
3. Surman, O., Purtilo, R. 1995. Re-evaluation of organ transplantation criteria: Allocation of scarce resources to borderline candidates. In Thomasma, D., Marshall, P. *Clinical Medical Ethics Cases and Readings*. New York: University Press of America.

4. Daniels, N., Light, D., Caplan, R. 1996. *Benchmarks of Fairness for Health Care Reform*. New York: Oxford University Press.

5. Dougherty, C. 1988. *American Health Care: Realities, Rights and Reforms*. New York: Oxford University Press, pp. 3–34.

6. Committee on Doctrine of the National Conference of Catholic Bishops. 1995. *Ethical and Religious Directives for Catholic Health Care Services*. Washington, DC: United States Catholic Conference.

7. Rawls, J. 1971. *A Theory of Justice*. Cambridge MA: Harvard University Press, pp. 54–114.

8. *United States v. Holmes*. 1842. 26F Case 36 (No 15, 383) C.C.E.D. Pa.

9. Rescher, N. 1969. The allocation of exotic medical life-saving therapy. *Ethics* 79(3):173–186.

15

Compensatory Justice: Social Sources of Claims for Health Care

Objectives

The student should be able to:

- Distinguish between distributive justice and compensatory justice.
- Define "accident" and describe how the notion of accident is relevant to questions regarding compensatory justice.
- List several examples of accidents.
- Identify a range of policy options that could be adopted in situations in which compensatory justice is being considered as an appropriate response to harm.
- Describe some cautions that should be taken into account when compensatory justice issues are being considered.

New Terms and Ideas You Will Encounter in This Chapter

Compensatory justice
Accident
Worker's compensation

Labeling
Social justice

Topics in This Chapter Introduced in Earlier Chapters

TOPIC	INTRODUCED IN	DISCUSSED IN THIS CHAPTER ON
Distributive justice	Chapter 3	Page 274

Introduction

Justice issues often are difficult to grasp because they require us to move beyond the usual one-on-one situation of health care interaction and consider whole groups of people. In Chapter 14 you began your inquiry into the questions of justice, so you know what I mean.

In this chapter I add a complicating but interesting dimension to justice that will be pertinent in some of the situations you will face as a health professional. The issue of compensatory justice often (but not always) is raised in situations in which people have health problems related to what Michael Walzer calls "hard work."

> [Hard work] . . . describes jobs that are like prison sentences, work that people don't look for and wouldn't choose if they had even minimally attractive alternatives. This kind of work is a negative good, and it commonly carries other negative goods in its train: poverty, insecurity, ill health, physical danger, dishonor and degradation. And yet it is socially necessary work that needs to be done, and that means that someone must be found to do it.[1]

The story of the Maki brothers will help you focus on how the issue arises in the context of patients' work and also as a means of helping you to think about other contexts in which compensatory justice considerations arise. It is more lengthy than some of the other stories:

THE STORY OF THE MAKI BROTHERS

Mr. Eino Maki is an asbestos miner who emigrated from Finland to the United States in 1945. He was born into a poor rural family who lived in a small village near the Russian border. Eino did not attend school in Finland after the first grade. In the village school he was ridiculed because of a speech impediment and facial disfigurement from a cleft palate. His family was too poor to send him to a special school in Tampere, some 300 miles away, and they needed his help on the farm.

During World War II the family farm was destroyed. Eino and his sister were sent to live with an aunt and uncle in Helsinki. After the war, at the age of 18, he could not find work in Helsinki, so he emigrated to the United States to live with his unmarried older brother in an area where there are many asbestos mines. The community there is about 90% Finnish.

Upon arriving in the United States, Eino went to English language school but had great difficulty both with his written and spoken language skills. After 3 months of agonizing attempts, he gave up. Today he speaks only a little English, and that is difficult to understand. He has basic reading and writing skills, at about the level of a first-grade student.

When Eino arrived in the United States, his brother John attempted unsuccessfully to find him a job in the railroad construction company where he was employed as a section worker. After several months Eino did secure a job in a nearby asbestos mine.

He has been employed by this same mining company and has held essentially the same position for the past 36 years. Although at work he still suffers the stigma associated with his cleft palate, he does participate in the social life of the community. Many evenings are spent reminiscing about the "good old days" in Finland, and everyone talks about going back. Privately, however, John and Eino agree that it is unlikely they ever will return.

In the past two or three months Eino has had increasing difficulty breathing. Occasionally he has coughed up blood-tinged sputum and often has pains in his chest when he awakens, but they disappear after he has been up and around for a couple of hours. At first he doesn't say anything to John, but one November morning he realizes that he can't make it to work. He asks John to take him to the company physician.

Eino has never liked doctors. In 36 years of employment he has visited the company physician only for the required routine physicals and once when he suffered a dislocated shoulder in a fall from a mine platform.

After the examination the physician assistant who has conducted the initial tests tells Eino that some further tests are needed and that he will have to be admitted to a hospital about 120 miles away. Eino is angered at this news but realizes that he cannot go back to work feeling the way he does. He tells John he wants to rest at home until he feels better, but John urges him to go to the hospital and drives him there.

Five days later in the hospital Eino takes a sudden turn for the worse. John is called and drives back to the hospital. When he arrives he is met by Dr. Nielson, a young physician who looks to John as if he can't be a day over 16 years old. Dr. Nielson asks John to come with him to a little room next to the nurse's desk and closes the door. "I'm afraid I have some bad news," he says. "Your brother has cancer and has had it for quite a long time. Ideally we would start a type of treatment that the company health care policy will not totally cover."

So far John has barely been hearing what the young doctor is saying. His mind is racing wildly. He vaguely recalls a discussion at a union meeting a year or so ago regarding a rumor that work in the asbestos mines causes cancer and that their union was looking into it. He had tried to raise the issue with Eino then, but Eino brushed it aside, said it was "a bunch of hogwash," and refused to discuss it further. John thought that Eino probably didn't know anything about it because although he was a loyal supporter of his union, he seldom attended union meetings. John let the matter drop.

Finally, John realizes that Dr. Nielson has been talking to him. "We could do the treatment, but unless Eino has additional insurance coverage, it is going to cost him a lot of money. Maybe he'd have to sell his house or use up whatever savings he has."

John tells the physician that they own a small cottage together, with about two acres of unfarmed land around it. They have no savings. Dr. Nielson replies, "Well, for Eino to receive the required therapy you may have to sell that house, Mr. Maki. Once you have expended your own holdings, you will be eligible for federal assistance. Of course, we can't guarantee that the treatment will beat the disease, but we feel reasonably sure that it would at least slow down the rate of growth of the cells."

There is a pause. Then he adds, "It is, of course, a big decision. It is entirely up to you and your brother what you decide to do. We haven't talked to him or rather been able to talk to him. He doesn't like doctors much! Why don't you talk it over, and I'll ask the social worker to spell out some of the details. Remember, it's your decision and your brother's. But don't take too long in deciding. . . . I think every day counts. Also, if you still have questions after talking with the social service department, have them set up an appointment for you to see me again."

As John stands, Dr. Nielson extends his hand and shakes it warmly. John glances up into the doctor's face and sees an expression of genuine pity in the young man's eyes. John blurts out, "Was the cancer caused by the mines?" The young doctor drops John's hands and studies his own hands as he answers, "Mr. Maki, the cause of cancer is often complex. It can be the result of a combination of factors. But the type of cancer that your brother has is the same type that asbestos miners get at a higher rate than the general population. Primarily it affects the lungs."

John thanks Dr. Nielson. Outside the doctor's office he wanders over to a window and stares outside into the snowy darkness for a long time, his hands in the pockets of his overalls. He has never cried since their brother Matt was killed in a tractor accident many years before, but he feels a lump rising in his throat now. He feels totally unable to move, as if he is glued to the floor. He struggles to think clearly, but his mind remains a blank.

The story of John and Eino Maki raises numerous ethical issues, most of them related to the justice of what has happened to Eino Maki and, more importantly, to what happens to people like him in our society.

DISTRIBUTIVE AND COMPENSATORY JUSTICE

The question of distributive justice, discussed in Chapter 14, is present here as an issue. People in situations such as Eino finds himself experience medical need, and from the way Dr. Nielson talks, there is some hope of palliation if the "ideal treatment" is made available. If treatment is justly distributed to each according to his or her medical need, there should be a way for the Einos of the world to receive the treatment. In this regard the inability of Dr. Nielson to initiate treatment on his own indicates that he himself is a victim of "the system."

The complicating factor is that payment is required for treatment. There is treatment available for persons like Eino if they can pay for it or render themselves financially impoverished enough to become eligible for government funds. And so in a case such as this the real criteria for receiving treatment is not only that a person shows need for a medical treatment but also that he or she has the resources to pay for it. In Chapter 14 you learned that this is distribution based on _____ and need. (If you answered "merit," you are correct.) In short, such a person will receive treatment because his treatment costs will be covered.

As a question of justice, however, Eino's situation is most perplexing not as a distributive justice issue but rather as one of compensatory justice.

Compensatory justice concerns compensations for wrongs that previously have been done. The compensation is not necessarily for a consciously perpetrated wrong. Even in the case of a person who is wronged by "accident," there may be an appeal to the concept of compensation to help rectify the wrong.

What does it mean to be harmed by accident? Try to think of some examples and jot them down here before proceeding.

_____

_____

Now read on:

The term *accident* can signify any situation a person could not have avoided but by which the person is harmed. It is the opposite of a situation that a person willfully and consciously brings into being and that could have been avoided. The following are some examples of an accident:

1. Being injured in a car accident that wasn't your fault
2. Being born and raised in an inner city ghetto
3. Being mentally retarded
4. Being in a job that is valued by people in society but that carries with it fatal or debilitating medical conditions that were not known at the time one accepted the position
5. Being a person who contracts cancer because of a medication one's mother took during pregnancy

The important point common to all these examples is that one cannot blame the person for his or her predicament.

In Eino Maki's case the accident that we are most concerned with is example 4. As far as we know, up until the time his brother John approached him about it, Eino had no inkling that his job might cause cancer, and it is likely that the cancer already was present by then anyway. In other instances, negligence or even outright malevolence can be found as the cause. But whether the result was consciously perpetrated or an accident, in each instance ascribing blame somewhere or to someone does not necessarily rectify the situation from a moral point of view. It must be asked what more, if anything, is morally required.

COMPENSATION AND COMPANY POLICY

The compensatory justice issue arises in the form of trying to decide whether Eino and those similarly situated ought to be compensated for the harm that has been done them, regardless of whether anyone is really to blame for it. The issue can be discussed by comparing several policies that might be adopted by companies, governments, or other policy-making bodies.

As you read these alternatives, try to think about which one(s) you could support and why:

1. The company should offer Eino (and all similarly situated employees) a sum of money equal to that which would pay for the treatment and provide early retirement with all retirement privileges if the person is unable to return to work. It is up to the affected employee to decide whether to spend the money on treatment or something else.

   Support _____ Don't support _____

   Reason(s) _____

2. The company should pay for the employee's treatment with the understanding that he or she will return to work if medically able and, if unable, will be retired with full privileges.

   Support _____ Don't support _____

   Reason(s) _____

3. The company should pay for the employee's treatment with the understanding that he or she will return to work if medically able. If unable, the person will be terminated with whatever retirement and other privileges have accumulated to the time of discharge.

   Support _____ Don't support _____

   Reason(s) _____

4. Federal legislation should be passed that provides Eino (and all similarly situated people) a sum of money from tax dollars equal to that which would pay for the treatment and arrange to supplement his retirement earnings up to his company's full retirement level if he is unable to return to work. It is up to the affected person to decide whether to spend the money on treatment or on something else.

   Support _____ Don't support _____

   Reason(s) _____

5. Federal legislation should be passed that allocates tax dollars to pay for full medical coverage for people like Eino but does not offer them a cash equivalent. That is, compensatory considerations have higher priority.

The understanding is that the person will return to the former employment if medically able. If unable, he or she will be retired by the company with full privileges, and the company will receive a subsidy from the government.

Support _____ Don't support _____

Reason(s) _____

6. No special allotment or allowances should be made for cases like Eino's.

Support _____ Don't support _____

Reason(s) _____

Options 1 through 5 all suggest that compensation ought to be provided for the wrong suffered by people like Eino Maki, although the form, amount, and source of compensatory funds differ.

The difference between a policy based strictly on the distributive justice reasoning discussed in Chapter 14 and one based on compensatory justice reasoning is highlighted by considering (1) the reasons beyond rights and medical needs offered for providing medical care coverage and (2) the resulting distribution of medical resources. As you read on, think about the policy options you have supported and not supported in your choices above, then continue to refine your thinking about which one option you can best support and why.

REASONS OFFERED FOR PROVIDING HEALTH CARE COVERAGE

In our discussion of distributive justice, medical need was proposed as the overriding reason for providing health care coverage (assuming that the medical condition is responsive to medical intervention). But in discussions of compensatory justice, natural or social conditions producing some type of victimized, undesired state become the overriding reason for providing medical care (or funds to pay for it). This type of reasoning is implied in options 1 through 5. To illustrate, in Mr. Maki's case the basic argument in favor of supporting his medical treatments financially is not that he has a terrible medical condition (which indeed he has) but that he has the condition *because* he was in a job that carried with it the albatross of carcinogenic agents.*

For many people examining Eino Maki's plight there is an intuitively sympathetic response in favor of compensating him for his supposed job-related cancer. It seems basically wrong, from a moral point of view, that he should have to suffer the ravages of a debilitating, painful, and fatal dis-

_____

*A carcinogen is a cancer-causing agent.

ease because unknowingly he has been working in a setting that carries a life-threatening hazard with it. (The additional important question of whether the company could have taken precautions and ensured the prevention of the condition would have to come into one's thinking about who, if anyone, is accountable for the situation. But even assuming that the company is innocent, the question of compensation can be raised as we are doing here.)

THE RESULTING DISTRIBUTION OF MEDICAL RESOURCES

In a distributive justice type of reasoning based on medical need, the more medically needy people take priority over those people whose needs are less pressing. It is taken for granted that all other characteristics of the people involved either are equal or have no moral bearing on the decision at hand. In compensatory justice reasoning it is possible that people with less pressing medical need but greater social disadvantage will have a greater claim on medical resources. Of course, in many instances a position of social disadvantage corresponds favorably with the degree of medical need, so that the resulting distribution looks the same. One cannot, however, count on the priorities being the same with the two types of reasoning. To think about compensatory justice you have to take into account whether Eino's being a poor immigrant forced by circumstance to spend his days working in a mine is a morally significant factor. A way of thinking about it is that he is shouldering more than his share of the societal burden simply by being in a position of doing the hard work of the society that Michael Walzer described in the introduction to this chapter. Almost all workplaces have an ethos that justifies rewarding people over and above others when their work is meritorious. A similar line of reasoning would move such people higher up on the scale of priorities for resources when they have medical needs equal to those of others.

One could argue that both types of medical problems (those caused by a medical condition alone and those in which medical need and other disadvantages are present) should be supported. I agree. But all too often there are practical limits on the overall resources, so that to do this would be at the price of some other, perhaps equally compelling, request. Compensatory justice is a position requiring us to reckon with the possibility that over and above medical need, there is an additional claim to resources by those whose need is related to social wrongs. The result of this position is that a duty to provide compensation modifies and overrides any general principle of distributive justice (i.e., based on medical need alone). Having considered all the ramifications so far, go back and choose one or two policy options you can best support now. Elaborate on your reasons:

Having read more about distributive and compensatory justice, I support option(s) _____ (and _____). My reasons are:

_____

_____

_____

Caveats Regarding Labeling

Although much can be said in support of compensatory justice, a practical difficulty must not be overlooked. Determining who among wronged groups in society will be singled out for preferential treatment requires that the people be designated as a special class. *Labeling* assures that already vulnerable groups become readily identifiable, often with accompanying labels. Such groups are not always given the preferential treatment promised them and may even be further discriminated against. For example, in the mid-1970s an extensive screening program for sickle-cell disease was initiated in the United States. Sickle-cell disease affects primarily African Americans. It is a painful condition manifesting itself in infancy and continuing throughout a shortened life span. Symptoms associated with it include infarction of the soft tissue and bone, causing acute pain. It also affects the spleen, liver, and kidneys.[2] The screening designed to identify affected individuals and therefore (it was implied) to offer them assistance has not been accompanied on a large scale by treatment programs that attend to their basic medical symptoms. Instead, in many instances African Americans identified through the screening process have found that insurance, employment, and other records carry stigmatizing information regarding their status as carriers of the sickle-cell trait. In short, people in a labeled group who have suffered previous social wrongs are not necessarily relieved of their afflicted position by policies that ostensibly singled them out for preferential treatment.

Private or Public Funds

An additional problem associated with this issue is determining who in the population should bear the burden of costs incurred as a result of policies based on compensatory reasoning. For example, options 1 to 3 suggest that the cost should be borne by the company. Implicit in these options is the idea that the company is somehow responsible for the injury (through inadequate safety measures etc.) or at least owes this caring response to a loyal member of the company "family" who through no fault of his own was struck down. These positions therefore require compensation solely in those cases in which accountability can be established.

Options 4 and 5 remove the condition of possible blame and more fully affirm that compensation for the harm itself is the decisive factor. Federal sources assume the cost through taxation of the population. Taxes come from those people who, under the United States doctrine of personal liberty, have been able to provide for themselves. Personal liberty is a value cherished by almost all members of our society. As taxes increase for the purpose of supporting individuals such as Eino Maki, the requirements of compensatory justice begin to impinge on the personal liberty of people who are not ill or presently in need of medical services. They cannot send their children to colleges they otherwise would choose, put additions on their homes, buy sports and exercise equipment to keep fit, or, for some, heat their homes properly.

To arrive at a policy, the question is how much personal liberty a society is willing to sacrifice to uphold justice.

Even when the issue is not put into the federal policy arena and remains at a local policy level or the level of private insurance, the concerns are similar. If the people involved belong to private plans, the premiums continue to go up, taking more and more of the gross earnings of individuals.

Having considered all the ramifications, suppose that you are a member of a policy-making body that must vote on policy options 1 through 6. Of all the options, which one will you support now? Option _____
Why?_____ _____ _____

_____ _____

Even though you have been a responsible committee member and have supported what in your judgment is the best option, what (if any) lingering reservations do you have regarding your choice? _____

In making this policy decision you have exercised your moral reasoning in a manner similar to that which you will be asked to use in the practice of your profession. Although the emphasis in this exercise has been on the options, in your process of coming to a decision you also have had an opportunity to consider the relevant facts, bring to consciousness the dilemmas or distresses your choice creates for you, consider the type of person you want to be, and focus on a weighing of either duties or consequences. Having acted (by voting) you have successfully engaged in five of the six steps of ethical decision making introduced in Chapter 5. To complete the task, you will reflect on your decision and action afterwards.

SOCIAL JUSTICE AND THE PATIENT'S RESPONSIBILITY FOR HEALTH MAINTENANCE

The story of Eino Maki raises important questions about how to allocate scarce resources when some people in society are more disadvantaged than others because of their social situation. Eino was a hard working miner, and at least some people who read his story probably are sympathetic to him. Today there is a lively discussion about how the social responsibility to allocate resources justly can be balanced against each person's responsibility to try to stay as healthy as possible. The weighing of various determinants of claims is the work of *social justice*. The story of Jane Tyler and Sam Puryo illustrates some of the complexities that arise in the process of trying to exercise justice for everyone in a society. She too has life-threatening cancer, but her situation also is different from Eino Maki's in some striking ways:

THE STORY OF JANE TYLER AND SAM PURYO

Jane Tyler, a 32-year-old single woman and mother of three children (ages 5, 8, and 12), has been living on public assistance since her first child was born. Jane lives with her mother, who helps with light housekeeping and child care. Now that the children will be in school she has successfully applied for a grant that will allow her to train to become a physical therapy assistant so that she can make a living for herself and her family. Receiving this award was a tremendous boost to her self-esteem, and she sees it as a bright doorway out of her "no exit" life situation.

Therefore it comes as a devastating blow to her to learn that she has lung cancer. She has been threatening to stop smoking for a long time, but her two-pack-a-day habit has had a strong grip on her. It is an even greater shock to learn that although the cancer has not yet metastasized, she may not be eligible for state-of-the-art curative treatment because she is on public assistance. It seems that the state legislature presented to the voting public the opportunity to decide priorities for high cost interventions provided through public funds by sending a questionnaire to a sample group. The public sample of taxpayers eliminated from the list of priorities "debilitating or life-threatening disease clearly caused by smoking" (as well as many other conditions). Three physicians have concurred conclusively that Jane's type of cancer is caused by smoking. One of them believes there may be cofactors that lead some people to actually get cancer while others do not. The other two are completely convinced her smoking directly has created the health problem. As only two concurring physicians are needed for this policy to take effect, she is unable to receive the state-of-the-art treatment. Her only opportunity for the new treatment is for her to find some way to pay for it.

Sam Puryo is a social worker who has been Jane Tyler's case worker for several years. He is upset at what he judges to be the apparent injustice of the laws that have put her in her present predicament. He tries to call his state senator to see if there are any loopholes in the law that could help her or if an exception can be made for this woman who Andy sees as exceptional. The senator is not encouraging: She is sympathetic but knows of no loopholes and is pessimistic about an exception being made for anyone.

During a coffee break, Sam gets into a discussion of the new rulings with another social worker and other colleagues. His fellow social worker is strongly in favor of the approach taken by the legislature. All the people at lunch agree that it is important to be willing to consider the arguments.

As you have already learned, justice has been defined in various ways, each of them based on the fundamental idea of giving to each his or her due. But the following questions must be raised: What is due Jane Tyler and other people in situations like hers? More important, How should her situation be approached to ascertain what is due her ethically? Before proceeding, jot down your thought in response to these questions:

There are at least three variables that might be relevant in trying to sort out your answer: One is her medical need. A second is her low economic status, and the third is her apparently self-inflicted condition.

The first, her medical need, was introduced in Chapter 14 as being relevant from the point of view of distributive justice. In this approach, all people are seen as equal and therefore deserve equal treatment except when departure from such treatment is justified by relevant criteria. The distinctions of merit, ability, contribution, and need are intended to make possible the just distribution of limited human and material resources. In clinical decisions the criterion of need is considered decisive. Therefore if I were looking at Jane's situation strictly from a distributive justice stance, I likely would conclude that the medical care is due her strictly on the basis of her medical need.

In this chapter, however, you were introduced to the idea of justice based on the idea of compensation. It is called compensatory justice because it attempts to approach what is due a person by thinking of compensating that person or group for previous harms that they have suffered. Looking at this from a compensatory justice standpoint we would have to consider Jane Tyler's poverty. In other words, her economic status may become another decisive variable in trying to figure out what justice requires in regard to her situation.

Why should she (or anyone who is poor) be "compensated"? In general, people who are born into poor or indigent families, regardless of their racial or ethnic heritage, have less opportunity to better their position than those who begin life with more financial stability. The novelist Charles Dickens, who so vividly portrayed the poverty in England during the industrial revolution, observed during an address to the Metropolitan Sanitary Association in 1851:

> If I be a miserable child, born and nurtured in the same wretched place, and tempted, in these better times, to the Ragged School, what can a few hours teaching that I get there do for me, against the noxious, constant, ever-renewed lesson of my whole existence?

Poor people are at a disadvantage in their opportunities to acquire an education and obtain employment that requires special skills or contacts, and women born into poverty are more economically disadvantaged than men. For Jane Tyler, poverty is compounded by gender. Besides lacking the educational and social advantages that would give her a better chance at financial security, as a woman, she also is limited in the job opportunities open to her. Finding an avenue to a skilled job such as being a physical therapy assistant could be an important turning point in her life and for her children's welfare. In short, one way to view Jane Tyler's situation is from the standpoint of compensatory justice only: She is poor; she is a woman. She has a "double whammy." In addition to needing basic health care, she deserves a high priority position rather than the lesser one she faces.

But now comes the further complication of her smoking-induced condition! You can see compensatory justice reasoning being applied again, but this time it is working against Jane Tyler. Most of us believe—in theory if not in practice—that most responsible citizens attempt to refrain from self-destructive behaviors. Now she is viewed tacitly, if not explicitly, as creating a harm through her carelessness and abuse, the harm being not only the destruction of her lungs but also the drain on tax monies required for her care. Do you think that she *is* voluntarily harming herself and others or is it an example of blaming the victim? What, if any, do you think are the difficulties in this approach toward Jane? Again, jot down your responses.

_____

_____

_____

One defining issue is whether in fact she is in a position to be held accountable for her smoking and the ensuing difficulties it has brought on her. Distinguishing between disadvantages that a person brings on himself or herself and those resulting from external forces over which he or she has no control is not easy to do. Some psychology theorists maintain that a person's conduct is determined in early childhood. Others believe that a person can be held accountable for every action he or she takes—that is, that even insanity is in some way chosen and therefore does not relieve one of responsibility for one's actions. What do you think?

_____

_____

_____

In health care this discussion and your responses are germane because many people feel that individuals ought to take more responsibility for their health.[3] According to their way of thinking, someone who has liver failure due to heavy alcohol intake would not be eligible for public aid for health care services because the disease results from his or her chosen lifestyle. But there is also great risk of injustice in such a strict accounting, for our knowledge about the determinants of alcoholism is still quite limited. In addition, one could argue that the alcohol-dependent person is a victim of an unfavorable social status, unhappy childhood, or psychiatric disorder.*

Although we cannot help but have opinions and personal feelings about issues related to justice, it is important to remember that the relevant arguments are usually general, not specific. If public funding should be available for any disadvantaged person, then it should be available to all those who need it. One philosopher has set out a general rule for the consideration of this problem. He proposed that "All primary social goods . . . the bases of self-respect—are to be distributed equally unless an unequal distribution of any or all of these goods is to the advantage of the least favored."† How you will respond to these various viewpoints in regard to health care resources depends in part on your idea of justice. If departures from allocations for identical medical treatment must be based on medical need alone, your answer will be different than if medical priorities should also be based on the greater general (e.g., economic) status considerations of some people in society and their ability to take control over their own destinies.

In short the issue of public funding for health care is one of many in which both distributive and compensatory justice principles have been upheld as relevant. Do they conflict? Does one supersede the other? According to compensatory justice, disadvantaged people should receive a higher priority in regard to their health care needs (including treatment of self-induced, health-threatening conditions). As an emerging professional your generation will be on the front lines of determining the extent to which Western democratic societies determine to care for their own, even those who cannot pay for their basic health care services.

SUMMARY

The issues raised in this chapter admit of no easy answers, theoretically or in their practical application. It is to be hoped that you will have time to reflect on the implications of such policies and think through the advantages and disadvantages of the options. Especially worthy of consideration are the problems that arise when the criteria for determining health care priorities move beyond that of clinical need. The challenge to all is to discern

---

*For moral missteps due to your own feelings about persons with characteristics such as these, see Chapter 13, The "Difficult" Patient.

†From *A Theory of Justice* (p. 3) by John Rawls. Copyright © 1971 by the President and Fellows of Harvard College. Reprinted by permission of Harvard University Press.

when it is morally defensible to allocate these resources according to other criteria and, in so doing, prevent an arbitrary elitist system of distribution.

Questions for Thought and Discussion

1. Some have argued that because the extent to which people value health in relation to other goods (such as food, shelter, clothing, a car, living where there is fresh air, etc.) varies from person to person, the most just health care resource distribution would be to give the same amount of money to each citizen and let him or her spend it however he or she chooses. Discuss the strengths and weaknesses of this arrangement.

_____

_____

_____

_____

At what age should this allocation be made? Why?

2. Discuss the pros and cons of the following situation from the point of view of compensatory justice considerations. Condition A is a progressive, debilitating disease of the central nervous system. It first affects the spinal cord and in its later stages infiltrates the brain, resulting in progressive spasticity and later in multiple movement and thought disorders. It occurs primarily in white middle-class men 40 to 55 years of age and leads to certain death in 15 to 20 years.

The cause and course of the disease is well understood. It is an autoimmune condition. Recently a medication has been discovered that can help to slow the progress of the disease dramatically. At present, however, the cost of the medication required for treatment is estimated to be about $10,000 per year for each patient. About 750 people in the United States have been diagnosed with the disease, and the incidence seems to be increasing. It is believed that many more cases may surface if the medication becomes available for any who need it.

Legislation has been introduced into the U.S. Congress to make possible the processing and administration of the drug "in the name of humanity." A conservative estimate is that the cost to U.S. taxpayers will be about seven million dollars per year.

When the bill is being discussed, a counterproposal is introduced by a group representing Latinos. They propose that the money be spent to provide full dental care, free of charge, to any Latino child in the United States up to twelve years of age whose parents earn less than $6000 per year. Although some are able to pay for dental services, their argument is that most are not. The cost, according to their estimate, will be about equal to the treatment program being proposed for condition A but will serve about ten times as many United States citizens. The core of their argument is that in general the Latin American individual has been discriminated against in the United States and that legislators and policy makers must take this factor into account in determining health care priorities.

References

1. Walzer, M. 1983. Hard work. In *Spheres of Justice*. New York: Basic Books, pp. 165–183.
2. Purtilo, D.T., Purtilo, R.B. 1989. Inherited diseases. In *A Survey of Human Diseases* (2nd ed.). Boston: Little, Brown, pp. 295–297.
3. Brody, H. 1995. Patients' responsibilities. In Reich, W. (Ed.). *Encyclopedia of Bioethics*, rev. ed. New York: Macmillan, pp. 1921–1923.

16

Living Ethically within the Organizations of Health Care

Objectives

The student should be able to:

- List three areas addressed by "organization ethics."
- Define "mission statement" and the role of mission statements in the organization life of contemporary societies.
- Describe what policies are and what they are designed to accomplish within health care and other organizations.
- Discuss several ethical elements that can be applied to an assessment of whether a policy is based on sound moral footing.
- Describe what it means for individuals to have a prima facie obligation to honor policies.
- Identify some ways in which the utilitarian approach to health care organization policy serves everyone well and conditions under which serious shortcomings may arise from relying on this approach.
- Identify three obligations that organizations have to individuals.
- Name some virtues of organizations and why they are important in today's evolving health care system.
- Critique key policies and administrative practices in the health care institution where you are training.
- Describe four areas in the business and management of an organization that require ethical reflection.

New Terms and Ideas You Will Encounter in This Chapter

Organization ethics	Standardized protocols
Business ethics	Mission statement
Managed care	Policies
Capitation	Cost-effectiveness

Topics in This Chapter Introduced in Earlier Chapters

Introduction

An emerging area of ethical reflection in health care is organization ethics. *Organization ethics* pays attention to the values and duties expressed in the

- mission statements,
- policies and administrative practices, and
- business priorities

of institutions that deliver health care, government bodies that regulate health professionals and health care practices, professional associations, and profit or not-for-profit enterprises that own or manage health plans. These entities concerned with the larger social and bureaucratic organization of modern health care have goals that are not limited solely to the ethical goals of health professionals. At the same time none of these other goals necessarily is unethical either. For instance, a business goal of increasing the profit margin each year is legitimate for the type of entity a business is. *Business ethics* addresses the *conditions* under which a profit can be ethically realized and the *amount* of profit that is acceptable for the type of services. The overall goal of business, however, is to make money, which in itself is not wrong. As a member of a health care organization your challenge is to assess whether organization values and duties affect your professional practice positively or negatively when measured against the standard of your professional values and duties. Recently in the United States the ethical impact of organization behavior has become a focus of attention because of managed care. Managed care brings together the delivery and financing of health care services. Practices such as *capitation*, which limits the amount of care a whole group of similarly situated patients may receive, have caused professionals to reflect seriously on what such an arrangement means for each patient. The organization develops or adopts a *standardized protocol* for all patients who have similar clinical problems. The protocol determines what treatment each patient will receive. If an individual patient's care is not compromised by the protocol, the resulting cost savings corresponds favorably to professional ethics standards. If quality is cut for the purpose of a larger business profit, professionals should resist the practice.

In short, a health professional may be faced with an ethical problem in response to a sound business practice. Challenges also may arise in response to a mission statement, policies and administrative practices, and larger societal interests.

In the next few pages these areas of organization ethics will be described to give you an opportunity to think about your role in response to some issues that may arise. Most of the focus of this chapter is on policies and administrative practices because they are the areas where you will most directly feel their effects and where you will have the greatest opportunity for being change agents when necessary.

LIVING WITH MISSION STATEMENTS

A *mission statement* is an institution's or professional organization's brief description of its ideals and aspirations. Because the mission statement is stated in general terms, the employee often ignores it completely when joining the group. It is from these ideals and aspirations, however, that goals, behavioral objectives, and expectations of all users (e.g., patients and all employees of a hospital or other health care institution) are derived. Like codes and oaths, mission statements are public statements designed to declare to all the type of organization it is. Sometimes the values of the entity are reflective of religious assumptions. In the United States there are many hospitals and schools owned and operated by religious groups, a situation visitors to other parts of the world may not see. Such an organization will make reference in its mission statement to its understanding of the relationship of humans to God and each other and to the way in which the organization views itself as participating in the larger cosmic and social scheme of things. An example of a mission statement is shown on page 286. What can you tell from reading it?

What does this document tell you about the nature of this institution?[1] What does this document not tell you? To what audiences do you think it is directed?

Mission Statement
Saint Joseph Hospital is committed to the prevention of illness,
the restoration and improvement of health,
and the compassionate care of the suffering.
We are dedicated to the preservation and enhancement of life
by providing leadership in patient care,
education, and research
responsive to the health needs of our community.
We will pursue our vision
with the Judeo-Catholic heritage
as our foundation
and the hospital values
as our guide.

SAINT JOSEPH HOSPITAL
AT CREIGHTON UNIVERSITY MEDICAL CENTER

From Saint Joseph Hospital at Creighton University Medical Center, Tenet Healthcare Corporation, Omaha, Nebraska. Used with permission.

From reading it, what types of questions would you ask if you were seeking employment in this institution?

_____

_____

_____

What would you ask if you were new to this city and were trying to choose a hospital for your family?

_____

_____

_____

If you have not already guessed, the hospital is a Catholic hospital. You may have missed that it is also owned by a for-profit organization. Since mission statements become the basis for more specific policies and expectations, it is prudent as well as responsible to check the mission statement with as much care as you have read the St. Joseph Hospital statement before becoming part of an institution or organization. This check point will enable you to avoid ethical distress or dilemmas further into your affiliation with this body and its policies and practices if you do not subscribe to the overall nature of the organization's mission.

LIVING ETHICALLY WITH POLICIES AND ADMINISTRATIVE PRACTICES

Policies are statements designed to establish formal and informal guidelines for practice within an organization context. Policies should be consistent with the values of the entity. They should also be specific expressions of how the ideals in the mission statement can be carried out by the people in the organization as well as those the organization hopes to attract or serve. If policies are to be followed, they must also be clear, practical, flexible, and consistent with the values of the people or groups to whom they apply.

Today policies in health care reflect both traditional health care ethics and business ethics. As I heard one group whose mission was to deliver high-quality patient care comment, "No money, no mission." The goals of the organization often are not fully met simply by focusing on the model of a single patient and health professional. Fortunately for everyone involved, most administrative and business policies are sensitive to the demands for money and efficiency while not compromising the patient's well-being or the sanctity of the professional-patient relationship.[2] As you can imagine, however, the picture is not always rosy because an organization's policy may also come directly into conflict with professional ethics standards. In fact, it is often at the level of policy that goals for individual patients' well-being or justice among groups come into direct conflict with business interests. Recently I was conducting a workshop in a private health care facility that had adopted a "no AIDS patients" policy because of the high costs of services for many such patients. The health professionals were distressed because the facility was in the process of building a new multimillion dollar reception area and surrounding gardens with the hope of its beauty being the draw to "beat out the competition." This decision by the trustees of the facility was interpreted by my colleagues as being a triumph of profits over patients.

Few health professionals today will be in situations where they can ignore organization policies. Glaser maintains that partially because of the changes in the health care system, all ethical issues involving patient care now also have business-administrative and community dimensions. The three realms of ethics always are present.[3]

OBLIGATIONS TO HONOR POLICIES

Other sections of this book discuss your personal and professional values and duties in regard to patients, fellow team members, and yourself. A *prima facie obligation* to honor policies is an expression of your willingness to become a part of the larger environment in which your professional commitments can be met. (It has been a long time since you have encountered the term "prima facie duty or obligation." If you have forgotten what it means, return to page 60 for a quick review.) Without a posture toward policy that demonstrates your willingness to follow it, chaos could ensue, and even patient care could suffer dramatically.

When faced with a prima facie obligation to honor a policy, you should assess whether it is ethically supportable. One good test is to identify the purpose of the policy and also test it according to the ethical norms you learned in Chapter 3. You could ask,

1. Do the guidelines appear to encourage practices that will do more good than harm overall? If so, the policy could be supported from a _____ approach to ethics.

2. Is the policy aimed at preventing harmful discriminatory practices in the distribution of benefits and burdens? If so, it honors the principle of _____ .

3. Does the policy encourage respect toward everyone involved? Yes? Then it is consistent with the overarching duty to treat people with respect or _____ .

4. Does it allow some members to be rewarded for conduct that is exemplary in terms of improving patient satisfaction or employee morale or demonstrating good stewardship of environmental or other resources? If so, this policy encourages _____ .

5. Are the conditions of the policy imposed with appropriate consent and full participation of the involved parties and is the policy restrictive only to the extent it is necessary to protect some important value? If so, their _____ and the constraint required for the principle of _____ are at play.

If you filled in the blanks with

- utilitarian,
- justice,
- dignity,
- beneficence,
- autonomy, and proportionality,

you remembered well. If the policy supports these or other moral elements, you should be able to follow it with a clear conscience.

The obligation to follow policies is better understood in light of the fact that from the *institutional* standpoint an ethically supportable policy is the one that brings about the most good overall. (See No. 1 above.) Generally speaking, organizations have a utilitarian value system designed to provide the greatest good for the greatest number. It follows that from an organization standpoint, considerations of respect for individual autonomy may be submerged in favor of such utilitarian considerations as efficiency of operations and economic stability. Simply stated, the organization that fulfills its function of providing a worthwhile service efficiently usually is believed to justify the means employed to attain that end so long as the net result is a greater balance of benefits to humanity than would be realized if the organization did not exist. (For example, inadequate salaries could be justified by pointing to decreased costs to patients so long as the quality of their care did not suffer as a result.)

The idea of cost-effectiveness often is cited as the appropriate goal of health plans. The definition of *cost-effectiveness* is that the highest quality of care possible is provided at the lowest price. No one can argue with the underlying principle. The administrative arrangements, however, may succumb to the serious criticism that such efficiency can best be achieved through cutting costs by means that in the end actually compromise quality.[4] That, in fact, is the most serious criticism being leveled at many forms of managed care in which billing practices, access, financial incentives to health professionals, restricted access to specialists, shortened hospital stays, and other mechanisms designed to contain costs or improve profits are charged with denying patients *and* health professionals the consideration due them.[5,6]

Because policies invariably are generalities, they cannot provide the optimum solution to every situation. Often if they are made by administrators, they may be inappropriate or inadequate to handle every problem faced by a health professional. So policies merely provide boundaries. We all find ourselves breaking rules when overriding them can be justified, for example, parking in a No Parking zone to assist at the scene of an accident. That is, of course, why there is a prima facie but not an absolute duty to honor policies: What may be best for most people may not be best in a situation for a particular person.

OBLIGATIONS OF ORGANIZATIONS TO INDIVIDUALS

Policy in most organizations is established by those in powerful positions within the structure, although today multidisciplinary committees sometimes are assigned the task of designing, refining, and reviewing policy. In other words, today more and more people from all echelons of the organizational hierarchy are becoming involved in setting policy.

The Opportunity to Become Involved in Policy

Everyone should be given an opportunity to become involved in the policy process. The moral right of participation arises partly from the right to help determine those aspects of workplace practices that directly affect your well-being. Your involvement in policy development and review is the only way you can assure that you will not become caught in a situation in which you are forced to sacrifice important personal and professional values to the overriding organizational value of efficiency. Efficiency can be applauded when it can be brought in line with the professional values of faithfulness to patients, patients' and professionals' rights, and prevention of harm to anyone.[7] But only if concerned professionals are given—and take—the opportunity to become part of the policy development process will such coherence be the result.

A good place to start is your own place of employment or your professional association. Part of the ability to be involved in policy is to be able to ascertain where the policies are made and revised. Pertinent questions are

1. What is the name of the committee for a given policy process?
2. Who sits on the committee and what are their qualifications?
3. What must you do to be nominated for or appointed to the committee?
4. To whom must you speak to express your interest?

Students often get their start in shaping organizational structures by volunteering as student members of policy committees.

The Assurance of Relevant Policies

It is also reasonable to assume that your organization will have a range of policies and other administrative guidelines that give clear direction for your own practice. A health care institution devoted to direct patient care should have some or all of the following policies depending on the type of institution it is:

- Informed consent policy
- Withholding and withdrawing life-sustaining treatment policy
- Assisted suicide and euthanasia policy
- Advance directive policy
- Surrogate decision making, health care agents, durable power of attorney for health care, and guardianship process policies
- Do not resuscitate (DNR) policy
- Medical futility policy
- Confidentiality and privacy policy
- Organ donation and procurement policy
- Human experimentation regulations

- Conflicts of interest policy (including patient care and research policies)
- Admission, discharge, and transfer policy
- Impaired providers policy (including reporting procedures for impaired providers and medical errors)
- Conscience clause policy and procedures
- Reproductive technology policies

Can you think of others that would pertain to your professional responsibilities? If so, write them here:

_____

_____

_____

Obviously policies are not, in themselves, guarantees that ethical problems will be solved at the level of practice. At least four criteria, however, signal that the policy provides clear direction:

1. Consistency within the policy and the procedures that are developed to help implement the policy
2. A uniform method for resolving conflicts when various people affected by the policy disagree
3. Flexibility and a plan for a review of the policy
4. Education of everyone who will have to follow the policy[8]

Administrative Commitment to Creating a Humane Organization

Sincere and intense commitment to creating humane organizations is essential if those involved in the organization and the larger community are to thrive. Since most organizations are governed by a small number of people who have the final say over what will happen to everyone, this commitment must begin with the persons who have the most power and authority.

You already have learned that efficiency is one value of organization structures because they are designed to meet multiple needs and render multiple services. From a social standpoint, many would say that a "good" or "well-run" institution is an efficient one. From the standpoint of your tasks within a health care organization, however, you would benefit from institutions and systems that reflect virtues in addition to efficiency. Can you think of some? If so, write them down:

_____

_____

_____

John Rawls, a philosopher you have met before in your study of this text, has developed a provocative theory of justice as the primary moral trait or virtue of institutions.[9] He maintains that if an institution is fair in its assignment of rights and duties and makes provision for a fair distribution of its resources, then individuals in those institutions will be able to live more moral lives. Can you imagine what a courageous organization would be like and what type of policies and administrative guidelines you would find there? What about a compassionate or merciful institution? Philosophers, economists, and others maintain that institutions and other organizations do have character traits. They also acknowledge the power of organization structures to affect the lives of individuals in our highly bureaucratized society. The traits of health care organizations are one important focus of serious reflection today.[10] Underlying the concern is an awareness that modern societies have the capacity to fragment lives, alienate individuals from their values and connectedness, and marginalize already oppressed groups. Since so many people spend more time each week in the organizations of work, government, education, health care, and religion than they do in their own homes, all organizations must assume an influential role in helping to foster the moral life.

LIVING WITH THE BUSINESS ASPECTS OF HEALTH CARE

Business language often conjures up negative images of greedy health care institutions driven by profit at all costs. Although rare, such organizations do exist and, of course, create ethical dilemmas for health care professionals who work in them because they fail to meet reasonable expectations of patients and society. Not all health care institutions, however, are driven by a monetary bottom line. The business functions of any organization are designed to help meet the appropriate goals of that organization, whatever those goals may be. The business aspect of an organization primarily entails management related to advertising, hiring and firing of employees, establishment of policies and procedures, product or service management (design, production, and delivery), fiscal management, and operations.

Understandably, then, some major themes in business ethics are honesty in advertising and in dealings with partners and clients, fairness in the treatment of employees or others, criteria for quality control of the product or service, the meaning of fiscal accountability from the standpoint of taking everyone's legitimate interests into account, and the duty of respect for others in all the organization's interactions.

You can readily conclude some ways in which a health care organization such as a hospital, a nursing home, a home health agency, or an HMO would have to gear its business goals, policies, and practices to meet high ethical standards of patient care. At the same time it would have to determine how to maintain quality care while assuring fiscal stability and responding to the larger community's values and demands.[11] Good business also means creating mechanisms to assure the integrity of the system.[12] For example, billing practices that allow fraudulent charges for patient care reimbursement from insurance companies or through Medicare or Medicaid represent a system's failure in the structuring of appropriate checks and balances.[13]

Most management issues are brokered through policies and other guidelines. Organizations also have their own cultures, however, an ethos, habits, and informal decision-making mechanisms. Culture reflects attitudes about what is important, how the organization functions, and the incentives for certain types of behaviors.[14] To survive ethically within the organization where you work you will need to identify these business realities and critique them. Although it goes beyond the parameters of this book to address the business dimensions of your practice, the next generation of health professionals, to which you will belong, will be forced to be more cognizant of them. A firm grounding in professional ethics combined with the tools for ethical analysis you are learning here provide a basic foundation for this lifelong task.

SUMMARY

This chapter takes you out of the clinic or other immediate work environment and into the committee room and administrator's offices. As the complexity of the health professions and health care environment continues to grow, so do the necessity and opportunity for becoming involved in the development of mission statements, policies, and administrative and business practices. Such involvement should enable you to maintain professional standards and a high level of ethical practice. Despite the help that the organization policies, practices, and environment can provide, they are not an automatic guarantee of high-quality patient care or fair employee practices. You still must exercise good moral judgment about ethical problems.

Questions for Thought and Discussion

1. There is a moral dimension to the roles of administrator and health professional. The ethical priorities of each may differ and have bearing on the focus of policy. Using your own profession as a starting point, think of at least one point you and the administrator might want to include in a policy about accepting for diagnosis and treatment people who cannot pay for their care.

_____

_____

_____

2. List your own institutional obligations as a student or health professional and rank each one as having

   a. No ethical significance

   b. Possible ethical significance

   c. Definite ethical significance

   Which ones are determined by policies? Which policies?

   _____

   _____

   _____

3. Can you describe a situation in which you would consider a strike as an ethical action for yourself to take?

   a. If so, list the ethical issues pro and con.

   _____

   _____

   b. If not, why not?

   _____

   _____

4. Eudora Cathay has been a unit clerk at the same community hospital for two years. The position of unit clerk is a demanding one that involves answering the phone, relaying messages, coordinating laboratory personnel in their rounds, responding to physicians' requests, and making sure that patients are in the right places at the right times. Eudora's striking appearance is enhanced by her native African dress style. Some of the more conservative members of the staff, particularly physicians and administrators, have been disturbed by her style of dress. Others find it attractive and an interesting change from the wall-to-wall white uniforms everywhere in the hospital. The dress policy does not require unit clerks to wear a uniform and stipulates only that they be neat and well groomed (which she is) and dressed "appropriately" (which is controversial). Someone in an administrative position asked Eudora to dress more conservatively, and she refused on the grounds that she was neat and well groomed and any further demands were an invasion of her privacy. She was fired for her refusal to comply, amidst rampant rumors of racism. Discuss her situation in the light of good policy. Should there be a dress policy? Is there anything ethical about such a policy? Why or why not?

   _____

   _____

   _____

References

1. Mission Statement of Saint Joseph Hospital, Tenet Healthcare Corporation, Omaha, Nebraska. Used with permission.
2. Coy, J. 1993. Habits of thought: The community perspective. *PT Magazine*, July, pp. 74–75.
3. Glaser, J. 1997. Introduction. In Glaser, J., Hamel, R. (Eds.), *Three Realms of Managed Care: Societal, Individual, Institutional*. Kansas City, MO: Sheed and Ward, pp. vii–xiv.
4. Emanuel, E. 1997. Medical ethics in the era of managed care: The need for institutional structures instead of principles for individual cases. In Glaser, J., Hamel, R. (Eds.), *Three Realms of Managed Care: Societal, Individual, Institutional*. Kansas City, MO: Sheed and Ward, pp. 85–91.
5. Rodwin, M. 1995. Conflicts in managed care. *New England Journal of Medicine* 332(9):744–747.
6. Furrow, B. 1995. Managed care and the evolution of quality. *Trends in Health Care, Law and Ethics* 10(1–2):37–44.
7. Purtilo, R. 1988. Saying "No" to patients for cost-related reasons. *Physical Therapy* 68(8):1243–1247.
8. Miles, J. 1991. Responses to "From ethical dilemma to hospital policy." *Health Progress*, November, pp. 29–30.
9. Rawls, J. 1971. *A Theory of Justice*. Cambridge, MA: Harvard University Press.
10. Reinhardt, U. 1997. Wanted: A clearly articulated social ethic for American health care. *JAMA* 278:1446–1447.
11. Murphy, P. 1989. Creating ethical corporate structures. *Sloan Management Review* 81(Winter):81–87.
12. Hall, M. 1997. Bureaucratic and legalistic mechanisms. In *Making Medical Spending Decisions*. New York: Oxford University Press.
13. Woodstock Theological Center. 1995. *Ethical Considerations in the Business Aspects of Health Care*. Washington, DC: Georgetown University Press, pp. 4–12.
14. Copeland, L. 1995. Learning to manage a multicultural work force. In *On Moral Business: Classical and Contemporary Research for Ethics in Economic Life*, pp. 634–638.

17

Good Citizenship and Your Professional Role: Life As Opportunity

Objectives

The student should be able to:

- Describe two rights associated with having a career as a professional person.
- Compare the focus of "shared fate" and "self-realization" careers.
- Identify two ethical principles that apply to a health professional's duties to society.
- Recognize the difference between a professional's duty to promote service focused on the public interest versus the common good.
- Discuss at least two approaches to setting priorities that will better enable the health professional to be morally responsible.
- Reflect on how a basic respect for people may mean that the health professional will become involved in pressing social issues outside of health care.

New Terms and Ideas You Will Encounter in This Chapter

Good citizenship
"Shared fate" orientation of the professions
Right to work
Public interest versus common good considerations
Social responsibility

Topics in This Chapter Introduced in Earlier Chapters

TOPIC	INTRODUCED IN	DISCUSSED IN THIS CHAPTER ON
Responsibilities to Self	Chapter 7	Page 297
Rights	Chapter 3	Page 299

Introduction

Sometimes the health professional is involved in taking risks with dangers that are little understood. The little prince in Antoine de Saint-Exuperéy's famous children's story of that same name identified these dangers as "baobabs." This final chapter addresses the risks you may be asked to take as a professional person and a citizen with issues that endanger basic moral values of a society. In some ways you will have come full circle from the beginning of the book. There you were thinking about yourself first as a person. For instance, when we talked about responsibilities to self we were more concerned with how you could continue to develop your personal moral life as you assumed your professional identity and roles. Now we will start with you in the professional role and think about how it impacts you as a citizen.

Good citizenship is everyone's responsibility. The basic question, and an interesting one, is whether you have any *special* rights, duties, and responsibilities as a citizen because you are a professional. What do you think?

_____

_____

_____

To help focus your thinking, consider the following story:

THE STORY OF MICHAEL MERRICK

Two years ago the residents of Peetstown welcomed the arrival of ExRad Corporation. The town had suffered terribly when Cal Mode Textiles Corporation had left, and a major recruitment by the residents had resulted in ExRad's choice of their town for its new location.

Michael Merrick is a nurse in a rural health clinic in the northeastern United States near Peetstown. He grew up 10 miles from where he now works, although for several years he went to school and worked in New York City. He, his wife, and their three children moved here 4 years ago.

Recently Michael and his family went on a walk along the stream that flows through Peetstown. All of them simultaneously smelled a strong, sweet odor. John, the 10-year-old, ran upstream and discovered a small pipe just under the surface of the water. The odor was distinctly stronger in the pool that had formed there.

Michael suggested that they not go too near the water. They continued their walk. But that night he took a small jar and went back to collect a sample of the water. The next day he drove 40 miles to visit a chemist friend who works in a community college. The friend agreed to analyze the water and a week later called to say it contained large amounts of trichloroethylene, a toxic chemical that Michael remembered had poisoned the water supplying a town in Pennsylvania not long ago. Alarmed, Michael told the physician who visits the clinic biweekly about his findings. The two decided to pursue the matter by going to a county health official, who promised to take care of the problem. But a month went by, and Michael heard nothing. He tried calling the county official with no success. Finally he saw the man at the monthly Rotary Club meeting and asked him what was happening. The man took him aside and said, "Don't worry about it. It was nothing. The injection well belongs to ExRad Corporation, and they are looking into it." Then he added, "You know we need that corporation."

The next day Michael returned to the stream again. The odor was stronger than ever. When he got back to the clinic, he called the physician and related his story. She said, "I guess we had better pursue this ourselves, Mike." That night after dinner Mike discussed the matter with his wife. Both of them were worried about what lay ahead.

The ethical dilemma Michael and the physician face does not involve direct patient care, at least not yet. (We can imagine that the environmental hazard could cause illness down the road.) The threat of an environmental health hazard has come to their attention, and they must now decide what to do. What, if anything, do you think they should do?

_____

_____

Why? _____

Now that you have made an initial judgment, let us go through the story to highlight some basic ethical considerations. Then when the chapter is completed, you can see if you change your mind regarding the course of action they should take.

PROFESSIONAL AUTONOMY AND GOOD CITIZENSHIP

Professionals are a privileged group in society. In the first place they have had an opportunity to choose a career. Most of the world's population does not have such an opportunity. Having a career choice means that you are able to pursue your specific tastes, framing a life plan to suit your own character. Norman Care's classic paper on the nature of careers suggests that people in this privileged position choose between two basic types of careers, those with a *"shared fate" orientation* and those oriented to self-realization. The former focuses on service to society, the latter on self-satisfaction.[1] Health (and other) professionals fall within both categories to some extent, but primarily within the shared fate category, with its straightforward service ethic.

The *right to work*, whatever the job, is seen as a basic right in democratic societies. Work as a professional, however, is not a basic right for everyone. Depending on your profession, society will give you a license, which certifies you or registers you in the state where you work. Your right to work (as a professional) comes about only after you have completed rigorous training, passed qualifying examinations, and promised to adhere to the code of ethics of your chosen profession. All these hurdles are society's reassurance that you are competent to do what you "profess" to do.

A second dimension of your rights is your right to professional autonomy. The right to professional autonomy means that you have a right to use your skills to arrive at an independent clinical judgment about what is best for your patients or clients. Of course, as you have learned, the right to exercise independent professional judgment assumes that you have already gathered the relevant information from the patient, available to you through direct communication, surrogate decision makers, and advance directives.

Health professionals today sometimes are frustrated by regulations and policies that impinge on their freedom to exercise independent professional judgment. For example, you have encountered several examples in this book of managed care or government reimbursement forcing a patient to be discontinued from treatment too soon.

As you can probably conclude from this brief discussion of rights, a person who becomes a professional enjoys the same rights as other citizens regarding a right to work but also has the special, role-related right to act autonomously in making professional judgments. Of course, although this distinction is useful as a basic orientation to your place in society, it does not tell us much about how Michael should respond to his discovery of trichloroethylene in the stream or what he can reasonably expect from society in return for any activity he undertakes. To think about the ethical implications of Michael's discovery we need to address the further question of a professional's duties and responsibilities to society.

PROFESSIONAL RESPONSIBILITIES AND GOOD CITIZENSHIP

The traditional oaths and codes of professional ethics say little about the health professional's obligations to society at large, except as direct patient care can be viewed as having a positive impact on the health of the larger society. But modern codes and ethical guidelines almost always include such a focus. Check the code for your profession to see how this focus is worded and jot it down here:

_____

_____

Professional codes are often worded broadly to allow for further inter-pretation in more specific circumstances. Is this true of the statement you just wrote from your code? If you were using the statement as your guide, what would you do if you were Michael?

_____

_____

_____

You should now be aware that to guide your behavior you need to use some of the principles you learned earlier in this text rather than to rely solely on the code as a guide. Nonmaleficence will apply, as well as benefi-cence. Now the focus is society in general, not just an identified patient or client. Jennings et al.[2] distinguish two types of public service, each of which could be seen as meeting the criteria of nonmaleficence and beneficence. The first is service, which seeks to promote the *public interest*, and the sec-ond is that which promotes the *common good*.

> Public service that promotes the public interest includes the professions' contribution of technical expertise to public policy analysis, and indirect service to society that is a byproduct of service to individual members of society.
>
> Service that promotes the common good includes the distinctive and critical perspective the various professons have to offer on basic human values, and on facets of the human good and the good life. It also includes the profession's contribution to what may be called civic discourse . . . that ongoing pluralistic conversation in a democratic society about our shared goals, our common purposes and the nature of the good life in a just social order.[2]

This philosophical statement about the two types of service can be summarized as your responsibility to participate in the development of poli-cies and to address those larger social issues by which you may help to cre-ate a better society. As Jennings et al. put it, "the common good, therefore, refers to that which constitutes the well-being of the community: its safety, the integrity of its basic institutions and practices, the preservation of its core values."[3]

Of these two types of service, Michael's opportunity to pursue the prob-lem of the toxic waste being dumped into the stream more fully falls into the category of _____ _____ service. (If you answered, "com-mon good," you are correct.) Let's think about this more specifically. What are the important values that could be served by the involvement of Michael in this problem?

You probably agree that among the most important values is the safety of all living beings—the people, animals, and plants in the area—in other words the environmental health or general ecological balance. In recent years we have become more aware of the fragility of ecosystems and of the direct effects of imbalances on human health. Environmental or ecological illnesses are major sources of public health problems today.[4]

To think about how the health professions play a role in maintaining and restoring this type of health, health professionals should be seen as affirming a definition of health and well-being that goes beyond medical interventions strictly speaking. Michael's entering the public arena to prevent or remove harm to the whole community is as important as his interventions at the bedside.

SOCIAL RESPONSIBILITY AND GOOD CITIZENSHIP

Social responsibility involves all the ways in which you may feel that you should become involved in making the world a better place. To suggest that Michael is obligated equally by the broader public health and narrower clinical arenas raises the critical problem of setting priorities. In prioritizing the expenditure of your time and energies, fulfilling the professional obligations for which you are specifically trained takes precedence. After that you may choose to become involved in activities where you can be of assistance, even if you are not specifically qualified to do so. The least claim on you is made by activities in which you are less qualified than others to make a significant impact. This approach to setting priorities can be of great assistance when the tug of responsibility calls and you feel overwhelmed about choosing what to do and what to leave undone. You may find that the requirements of your job description do not coincide with your best judgment about where you can make the contributions that will matter most. This may be a call to reassess your vocation if you feel you have the freedom to make a change. At the very least, priority setting can give you a perspective from which to make important choices when the opportunity arises.

In considering Michael's opportunity, the first thing to decide is whether his pursuit of the toxic waste problem will deter him from performing his professional services, as these skills have the greatest claim on his time and energies. The second consideration is whether he should get involved at all (as a professional) in the toxic waste issue. He certainly could involve himself strictly as a citizen, but the question we are trying to explore is whether there is any professional duty to pursue it. In other words, from an ethical point of view the question is not may he, but should he?

I think that an additional useful approach to ascertaining his (and your) actual responsibility in such issues is suggested by Jonsen and Jameton. Although I first encountered this article many years ago, I find myself going back to it because it is so helpful. They divide professional and political responsibilities of health professionals into three general categories of suitability for an individual's involvement:

1. The most binding responsibilities are those directly related to patient care.
2. The second most binding are those related to the broader public health issues that all health professionals share.
3. The least binding are other opportunities for involvement.[5]

The third category, however, and this is key, will vary according to the health professional's judgment about how much difference her or his involvement might make on the basis of the health professional's "symbolic weight" in some types of issues. Sometimes a job is more likely to get done because someone of high status, respect, or visibility throws weight behind the issue. And so if Michael's status as a nurse (or health professional in general) will lend credence to the gravity of the offense or need for correcting the problem, his responsibility to get involved increases on that basis alone. Jonsen and Jameton also stress that although these are useful *general* guidelines, an urgent crisis may arise in which health professionals feel compelled to change the order of these responsibilities. An example was the physicians, nurses, and others who threw themselves into open resistance against the Nazi regime, placing the urgency of this social situation above all else.[6] The issue does not necessarily have to involve health care (although Michael's problem involves at least a public health issue). In short, if Michael is trying to set priorities, he will have to ask himself about the appropriateness of his involvement according to the three criteria of suitability.

What types of questions would you still need answered to decide whether Michael (and his physician colleague) should shoulder the burden of confronting a large corporation that is polluting the stream near Peetstown?

CARING—KEY TO GOOD CITIZENSHIP

Health professionals often find themselves faced with larger social issues that call for attention. Perhaps the best ethical framework for thinking about the rights, duties, and responsibilities of the professional as a good citizen is to set these principles within the larger framework of mutual respect and care introduced in Chapter 2. In Western cultures we often believe that because we want to act responsibly, we must carry the moral weight of an issue on our individual shoulders. Understanding our mutual interdependence allows us not only to call on our colleagues to resolve problems they are more suited to handle but also to count on their support when we are asked to share the larger burden. The boundaries of professional responsibility as such do not have well-defined edges, so that you may find yourself involved in a great variety of issues during your professional career. Working together with your colleagues, you can hope to have the energy, expertise, and wisdom needed to make a positive difference.[7]

An appropriate ending to the journey we have taken through this book together is to leave you with a famous quote from a great American novel, John Steinbeck's *The Grapes of Wrath*. It is a powerful literary statement about our interdependence and about the will to try to help fulfill high ethical goals. In this excerpt Tom has decided to join the ranks of people struggling against the injustices being perpetrated on the migrant workers:

> They sat silent in the coal-black cave of vines. Ma said, "How'm I gonna know 'bout you? They might kill ya an' I wouldn' know. They might hurt ya. How'm I gonna know?"
>
> Tom laughed uneasily. "Well, maybe like Casy says, a fella ain't got a soul of his own, but on'y a piece of a big one: an' then:"
>
> "Then what, Tom?"
>
> "Then it don' matter. Then I'll be all aroun' in the dark. I'll be ever'where: wherever you look. Wherever they's a fight so hungry people can eat, I'll be there. Wherever they's a cop beatin' up a guy, I'll be there. I'll be in the way kids laugh when they're hungry an' they know supper's ready. An' when our folks eat the stuff they raise an' live in the houses they build: why, I'll be there. See?"[8]

Tom has made the decision to be where there is suffering. That commitment may indeed take you into the heart of problem solving around issues that will not be resolved unless you "see" the difference your presence will make. I wish you well on this journey!

Questions for Thought and Discussion

1. Since you cannot become involved in every social issue that comes along, it is a good idea to choose the issues that hold some interest for you. If you were to become involved in trying to solve three social problems today, what would they be?

_____

_____

_____

_____

2. You have been invited to become a member of a state commission that will examine how to best use public space (parks, gardens, beaches, parking areas, etc.) for the welfare of the citizens. They have asked you because they think "your expertise as a health professional is needed." What do you think you could bring to such a commission from the point of view of your professional training and expertise?

_____

_____

_____

_____

3. Homelessness has reached momentous proportions. What can your profession do about the problem of people who do not have so much as a roof over their heads? What can you, personally, do?

_____

_____

_____

_____

References

1. Care, N. 1984. Career choice. *Ethics* 94(2):283–302.
2. Jennings, B., Callahan, D., Wolf, S. 1987. The professions: Public interest and the common good. *Hastings Center Report*, February (suppl):3–10.
3. Ibid.
4. Shiva, V. 1992. Recovering the real meaning of sustainability. In Copper, D., Palmer, J. (Eds.), *The Environment in Question: Ethical and Global Issues*. London: Rutledge, pp. 24–68.
5. Jonsen, A., Jameton, A. 1977. Social and political responsibilities of physicians. *Journal of Medicine and Philosophy* 2(4):376–400.
6. Rittner, C., Myers, S. (Eds.). 1986. *The Courage to Care: Rescuers of Jews during the Holocaust*. New York: New York University Press.
7. WHO Commission on Health and Environment. 1992. Health and the environment: A global challenge. *Bulletin of the World Health Organization* 70(4): 409–413.
8. Steinbeck, J. 1939. *The Grapes of Wrath*. New York: Penguin Books, p. 535.

Index

Page numbers in *italics* refer to illustrations; page numbers followed by t refer to tables.